Praise for *Superfoods*

"Imaginative . . . helpful and intriguing." —*Publishers Weekly*

"Virtually a course for smart eating, *Superfoods* is power packed with useful information and different, pleasing recipes . . . When a cookbook delivers the promise of its title, you know you have something wonderful." —*Lexington News-Gazette* (VA)

"Recipes are easy to prepare and offer plenty of variety—and even include heart-healthy meat entrees. In fact, they're so good you'll forget you're doing your body good." —*Longevity*

"The definitive handbook for the health-conscious who want great-tasting food . . . full of accessible and useful nutritional facts." —*Fancy Food*

"On target in a nutrition-conscious decade." —*Nation's Restaurant News*

"An essential tool for better living, this book is packed with information about vitamins, minerals and the disease-fighting qualities of particular foods." —*Women's Circle*

"*Superfoods* uses an encyclopedia approach to different foods and along the way tries to separate fact from fiction about their health benefits." —*The Star*

Superfoods for Life

250 Anti-Aging Recipes for Foods That

Keep You Feeling Fit and Fabulous

DOLORES RICCIO

HPBooks

HPBooks
Published by The Berkley Publishing Group
A member of Penguin Putnam Inc.
200 Madison Avenue
New York, NY 10016

First edition: February 1998

Published simultaneously in Canada.

The Putnam Berkley World Wide Web site address is http://www.berkley.com

Library of Congress Cataloging-in-Publication Data
Riccio, Dolores.
Superfoods for life : 250 anti-aging recipes for foods that keep you
feeling fit and fabulous / Dolores Riccio.
p.   cm.
Includes bibliographical references.
ISBN 1-55788-280-0
1. Nutrition   2. Longevity.   3. Cookery (Natural foods)
I. Title.
RA784.R498   1998
613.2—dc21   97-15698

Printed in the United States of America

1   3   5   7   9   10   8   6   4   2

Notice: The information printed in this book is true and complete to the
best of our knowledge. All recommendations are made without any guarantees on
the part of the author or the publisher. The author and publisher
disclaim all liability in connection with the use of this information.

For Rick, my love

Lucy, my daughter

and Joan, my friend

Contents

Acknowledgments

Many thanks to the special people who have believed in this book and helped to make it a reality: My husband, Rick, who tasted every dish and commented with loving discrimination; my friend Joan Bingham and my daughter, Lucy-Marie Sanel, who helped so much with the testing; Blanche Schlessinger, whose enthusiasm and resourcefulness are always inspiring; Jeanette Egan, whose knowledgable finishing touches have refined the manuscript; and John Duff, whose interest in the book from the beginning made it all possible.

Superfoods for Life

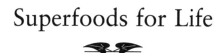

Introduction

NUTRITIONAL ELIXIRS FOR STAYING YOUNG

Growing older has never been richer in pleasant activities or more fulfilling in mature rewards than it is now. With so many happy possibilities in store, you know you have a lot of active living to do at any age. That's why nourishing your body and mind with the right foods, the superfoods, is not just important, it's absolutely critical to enjoying a good life— and a long life.

Most foods have some nutritional benefits, but those I have called "superfoods" have multiple benefits. They are the foods that offer the most vitamins, minerals, phytochemicals, and other important compounds that forestall aging and help you resist disease.

Your nutritional needs change with every passing year. The quality of your diet affects the quality of your life increasingly as time goes by. In every activity, from hiking a mountain trail to dancing all evening to starting a new business to writing a memoir, superfoods will help you to maintain the physical strength and mental power you need to live long with vigor and enthusiasm.

It's been estimated that one-third to one-half of the health problems experienced by people over fifty are related directly or indirectly to nutritional deficiencies. Some scientists have begun to think of the aging process itself as a disease of deficiency. Much of the degeneration that was once accepted as inevitable is now considered to be preventable for much longer than we ever imagined possible. Yet it's been found that people over the age of fifty often consume less than the Recommended Dietary Allowance (RDA) of some important nutrients: calcium, iron, zinc, copper, riboflavin, folate, and vitamin B$_{12}$. According to the National Eldercare Institute on Nutrition, one-quarter of older Americans have diets poor enough to border on malnutrition. Overweight also becomes more of a problem as lean body mass declines and body fat increases and is deposited in places we'd rather it weren't. This is because, beginning around the age of thirty, the metabolic rate starts to decline, altering a person's ability to balance food intake and energy needs effectively.

As much as you may need financial planning for your retirement years, you also need nutritional strategies for a long life. A nutritious diet can add five or more years to the average life expectancy at birth. More than following the latest fad in herbs or algae or chemicals or megadoses of single vitamins, it's the whole foods you choose to eat day after day that will most affect your health and allow you to continue to enjoy life's beautiful gifts of wisdom, love, creativity, and a rich spiritual philosophy.

Yes, We Can Outwit Nature

But we have to be knowledgeable to take advantage of the new realization that many of the undesirable effects of aging can be prevented; in fact, we have to outwit the negligence of nature. Once the reproductive cycles of the body begin to wane, nature seems to have less interest in keeping us in prime condition. No longer can we count on the resilience that nature pro-

vides so abundantly for the young. Immunity declines and cellular damage increases as years of living with pollution, pesticides, radiation, mental stress, and other hazards of the modern environment begin to take their toll. Before this happens, it's up to us to defend ourselves with important countermeasures—more awareness, more planning, more nutrients and phytochemicals to restore and rejuvenate us, and in some cases, even to reverse some of the aging process.

The superfoods in this book are the ones that have proven to be a first line of defense against continual degeneration, including the risk of diseases associated with aging: heart disease, cancer, adult diabetes, and cataracts, to name some of them. There are now literally hundreds of studies that suggest a diet rich in plant foods—fruits, vegetables, beans, and grains—decreases the risk of various kinds of cancer. It's been estimated that over half of the most common cancers are diet related.

The link between heart disease and diet was established much earlier, and the resulting change in eating habits must take some credit for the 23 percent decrease in death rates from cardiovascular disease that we have seen in the last decade. In a recent study of human subjects, called DASH (Dietary Approaches to Stop Hypertension), a diet of fruits, vegetables, low-fat dairy products, grains, and small amounts of fish and chicken, with a bottom line of only 27 percent calories from fat, lowered blood pressure in amounts comparable to drug therapy.

There are two population groups that have enjoyed a risk of heart disease lower than that of the rest of the world: the Inuits, who eat an abundance of oily fish, rich in omega-3 fatty acids, and the Mediterranean peoples, whose daily fare consists mainly of vegetables, grains, fruits, and olive oil. Following up on this, researchers in France tested a diet that incorporated both eating styles. After two years, the Mediterranean-plus-fish diet resulted in an incidence of heart disease that was 76 percent lower than that of the control group, which was were merely advised to eat less fat and cholesterol.

Mind—It Matters!

Along with defending against the assaults of bodily decline and diseases, superfoods also enhance your cognitive abilities—memory, reaction, and speech. When you consider that more than half of the 30 million Americans over the age of sixty-five are measurably brain impaired, protecting the brain with nutrition takes on a new importance. Superfoods supply the nutrients crucial to brain function [B vitamins, antioxidants, essential fatty acids, and minerals (iron, copper, magnesium, iodine, zinc, and boron)]. These help to prevent the accumulation of lipofuscin, a brown pigment that shows up on the skin as so-called liver spots and in brain tissue as senility. Many times what appears to be a mental aberration is ultimately traced back to a nutritional defi-

ciency. An inadequate supply of vitamin B_{12}, for example, causes neurological damage and sometimes mimics the symptoms of senile dementia. Even mental processes such as judgment and reasoning appear to be connected to high or low levels of various B vitamins circulating in the blood.

Researchers have discovered that people over sixty who have low blood levels of B vitamins and vitamin C score lower in cognitive tests than those with healthy vitamin levels. While cautious scientists decide which came first—did slower thinking lead to malnutrition or did malnutrition cause slower thinking?—it makes good sense to keep those vitamin levels high so that nothing will interfere with our enjoying the delights of the intellect.

There are superfoods that can help to relieve mental stress, which will enable you to cope better with the events that caused it. Certain foods stimulate the production of the neurotransmitter serotonin, your brain's natural tranquilizer. Other foods increase mental alertness when you need to be quick witted. It's important to know which ones they are and how to use them to best advantage. It's a very helpful strategy indeed to treat yourself to some tasty dish that will promote a desirable mental state.

Accentuating the Positive

"Today is the first day of the rest of your life" takes on more meaning with every year you live. The foods choices you make on a daily basis continually influence your future. But this is a *yes* book. Rather than worrying about what you should give up, accentuate the positive. Concentrate on these nutrition-packed superfoods and you'll just naturally eliminate the negatives of saturated fats and empty sugar calories—without feeling deprived. Build your menus around healthful dishes, cook them at home or choose them when you go out to eat, enjoy their lively good taste, and you'll be saying *yes* to your future years.

Age Doesn't Have to Make You Old

Everyone needs at least five servings of vegetables and fruits, including one of citrus and one of dark, leafy greens, as well as plenty of great grains and legumes on a daily basis. And the older you get, the more you need to be especially careful about getting enough of certain specific nutrients and phytochemicals among those servings, and here's why.

Current theory suggests that a major cause of what we call aging is the result of *free radicals* generated by the body's natural production of energy and by the stresses of exercise, pollution, solar rays, and traumatic events, physical or mental. A free radical is like a loose cannon on the deck. It's a highly reactive and unstable molecule that attaches itself to an available cell and even interferes with DNA. Free radicals can initiate a chain reaction that results in cancer. They can encourage the buildup of cholesterol and reduce our resistance to infection and disease. They can hinder collagen, which plays a role in keeping the skin looking young. If we could constantly and thoroughly cleanse the body of free radicals, it might be possible to take the "old" out of "old age."

The body has its own police force of enzymes to dispose of free radicals, but with advancing years, this force becomes less efficient than it used to be and needs the assistance of a knowledgeable nutritional boost.

Prescription for Feeling Fit and Fabulous

Nutritional researchers have found some energetic free-radical scavengers among the antioxidant nutrients that contribute substantially to the body's cell-protective system. These are vitamins A, C, and E, and the minerals selenium and zinc. Antioxidants have been shown to deactivate free radicals, fighting off degenerative diseases that are associated with added years. Antioxidant *foods*, rich in these compounds, appear to confer a better defense against free radicals than do antioxidant *supplements*. Whole foods, after all, not only carry the nutrients we know about, they also contain substances we have yet to discover. It's a generally accepted fact that supplements never contain all the health-building chemicals that foods do. There's actually a mix of about six hundred carotenoids and other vital nutrients in a diet rich in vegetables and fruits that may never be equaled by a pill.

As we age, the immune system gradually, silently, becomes less adept at warding off infections, some of which, like the flu, become increasingly dangerous in later years. You need to choose foods that will strengthen your body's ability to fight off the invasion of bacteria or viruses. Along with vitamins and minerals, defensive foods are also rich in protective phytochemicals.

Cardiovascular disease is the number-one health threat facing the longer-living population of today. Although most people are aware that diet has a vital influence on the cardiovascular system, often this factor is viewed from a negative angle, the *thou-shalt-not* school of nutrition. On the positive side, it's just as important to realize there are superfoods that will help to lower blood pressure, reduce cholesterol, lessen the risk of strokes, and preserve the potassium balance needed to guard against arrhythmias. These are the foods we want to maximize in our menus.

Super nutrition plays a role in defending our bodies against every kind of cancer, too, and there are many recent nutritional studies that have brought this good news to the attention of the scientific community. Researchers have discovered chemicals in foods that guard against the damage of carcinogens, or discourage the cell changes that result in cancer, or starve the progress of the disease. According to the American Cancer Society, a third of the country's cancer deaths are related to dietary factors.

Superfoods offer vitamins and minerals that preserve male potency as well as nutrients that guard against problems of the female reproductive system. Some of them are rich in the substances that avert certain kinds of birth defects. Others contain chemicals that protect against prostate disorders.

It becomes increasingly vital, also, to keep the digestive system in top working order with a sufficient amount of fiber. You also need to preserve bone strength by consuming not only calcium but also other nutrients that support a strong body.

Making the Most of Your Personal Best

As you add on birthdays, you may have cause to review certain predispositions in your genetic heritage or even have had your own share of health problems. Whatever challenges you've encountered, consistently emphasizing the superfoods in your day-to-day meals will boost your body's natural power to heal existing disorders and to avert recurrences—in other words, to be your healthiest self. Whatever your genetic weaknesses—and all of us have some—superfoods will help you contend with them. Good nutrition rejuvenates the life force, resists the onset of disease, and sometimes even reverses chronic conditions.

Feeding your body the fuel it needs is the basis and background from which you can proceed to other stay-well choices, such as physical activity, mental stimulation, emotional gratification, and spiritual seeking.

Superfoods Fit Your Changing Caloric Needs

With added years, alas, lean body mass (muscle and bone) decreases, while the proportion of fat increases, even though your weight may remain the same. Daily caloric needs drop by 10 percent each decade after age fifty, but your need for nutrients is greater. This dilemma is solved by *nutrition-dense* foods—the light, lively, lovely foods that have more nutrients per calorie by ratio than the heavy, stodgy, fatty, salty processed stuff. Consider, for example, cantaloupe: It's so rich in vitamin C, beta-carotene, and potassium and so low in calories that it definitely has more bounce to the ounce! Superfoods tend to be more nutrition dense than their counterparts. Compare, for instance, nonfat yogurt to sour cream. When you want to top a baked potato with something creamy, choose the yogurt with chopped fresh chives for more calcium and zero fat.

Choosing nutrition-dense foods has the secondary benefit of allowing you to consume a satisfying plateful of some really delicious foods without guilt. Eating, after all, is one of the joys of life.

Enjoy the Best Years of Your Life

Our middle years ought to be the prime of life, rich in the rewards of maturity, free of the urgencies and uncertainties of youth, and blessed with secure relationships. To enjoy the satisfactions and pleasures we've

earned through time, we need optimum good health, and the first step in that direction is to energize ourselves with the superfoods described in the following pages.

The Fun of Cooking Superfoods—and Some Practical Matters

Fresh, fast, and fun—that's what cooking superfoods should be. You'll find the recipes in this book are not only crammed with good nutrition but also easy to prepare, even after work. Healthy food shouldn't wait for the weekends!

Many of these recipes call for such cook's staples as chicken or vegetable stock. If you enjoy preparing a homemade chicken or vegetable stock, go to it! Recipes are given on pages 331 and 333. That's the best of all possible bases. But if time and energy do not permit such niceties, stock up on cans of a tasty low-salt alternative. It's also helpful to keep on hand various flavors of bouillon cubes as a backup; prepared bouillon can pinch-hit for canned broth.

All legumes are superfoods, and I've used them frequently in this book's recipes. Lentils, split peas, and fresh shelled beans cook in less than an hour, but other types of dried beans require presoaking and long cooking. Fortunately for the time-pressured cook, all types of beans are also available in cans. These useful products need thorough rinsing to rid them of gelatinous juices and excess salt, but they are a time-saving alternative. I suggest searching out a good, low-sodium organic brand, such as Eden, and keeping a supply of many varieties on your pantry shelf for quick inspirations. On the other hand, you'll find recipes for homemade dried beans cooked "from scratch" on pages 328–29.

Some of the whole grains called for in recipes may not be readily available in supermarkets, but they can usually be found in natural foods markets that feature organic foods. Bulgur (cracked wheat), whole-wheat couscous, brown basmati rice and other unrefined grains don't keep as well as their processed counterparts, but if you have space, most of them can be frozen for longer storage.

Herbs are always tastier fresh than dried. I find it both practical and pleasing to keep a few pots of fresh herbs growing on my kitchen windowsill in winter so that I can always put my hand on a few fresh sage leaves or thyme sprigs when needed. Fortunately, for those unwilling to cultivate a green thumb, supermarkets are increasingly offering bunches of fresh herbs all year. I do recommend buying these often, while still keeping a gardenful of dried herbs on your spice shelves. I find that fresh herbs, even parsley, keep best if treated like a bunch of flowers, with stems set in a small pitcher of water.

If you don't fancy a bouquet of parsley, another storage method is to stem and chop it, lay it out on a paper towel until it's somewhat dry, and then scoop the leaves into a jar. Refrigerated, the jar of chopped parsley should last until your next shopping trip. Fresh parsley is super rich in vitamins and minerals, as well as flavor. It's a breath freshener, too: One of the chief ingredients in one well-advertised over-the-counter internal breath sweetener is parsley oil. The culinary alternative is dried parsley, which is the least successful of all the dried herbs, having hardly any taste at all.

Forget the fear that a good tomato sauce needs hours of cooking and stirring. A basic tomato sauce is so easy to prepare (pages 321 and 325), you may never need to resort to buying it in jars again. Instead, stock up on cans of imported Italian plum tomatoes and the other makings.

The notion that some foods are better for you when not combined with others, or that fruits in particular should be eaten alone to avoid fermentation, is not founded in scientific fact. Foods eaten in nutritious, delicious combinations benefit from the synergy of their varied vitamin and mineral content. A good example is the mineral iron: Difficult for the body to absorb in its non-*heme* form (from vegetable sources), it's much more easily assimilated if a vitamin C–rich food is eaten at the same time.

The recipes in this cookbook were not written to be followed without variations. One leafy green vegetable or pasta shape often can replace another; onions can be used if shallots are unavailable; and if peaches at the market look better than the nectarines called for in a recipe, a little judicious substitution is always possible.

Healthful cooking should be easy and enjoyable so that you'll be encouraged to prepare and serve superfoods on a daily basis for a long, vigorous life.

The Anti-Aging Vegetables

Live longer and live better with these vibrant vegetables. Not only rich in free-radical-fighting antioxidant vitamins and minerals as well as defensive phytochemicals, vegetables also are a great source of fiber, which keeps your digestive system in good order. To get your recommended servings per day, you'll have to pack them in at lunch as well as at dinner.

An important category of vegetables deserves special attention. Known as *cruciferous* vegetables (from the Latin *cruc*, meaning "cross," because their flowers form a Greek cross with four petals), they contain indoles, sulphorafane, and other phytochemicals that protect against colorectal, stomach, and respiratory cancers by stimulating the production of enzymes that detoxify carcinogens. The evidence has been so compelling that the American Cancer Society especially recommends including this family of vegetables in your diet. Cruciferous vegetables include broccoli, brussels sprouts, cabbage, cauliflower, collards, kale, mustard greens, radishes, rutabagas, turnips, turnip greens, and watercress.

More good vegetable news in the beta-carotene category. People who eat more of those orange and dark green vegetables (and orange fruits, too) have a lower risk of many cancers. Included in this list are cancers of the esophagus, larynx, mouth, throat, pancreas, lung, colon, and bladder. No, you can't get the same thing from a supplement, as recent, disappointing tests have shown. How can this be? Researchers theorize that beta-carotene may be a marker for other phytochemicals and that the protective element may be the result of a team effort of all the elements involved in these foods. Synergy at work!

Heart disease and stroke are less likely among big vegetable eaters. Soluble fiber, potassium, and flavonoids are credited with this desirable development. And cataracts are less common among those who frequently dine on dark, leafy vegetables, because they're rich in lutein, a phytochemical closely connected to eye health.

So as your mother always advised, "Eat your vegetables!"

Artichokes—the Mediterranean Thistle

It takes time to eat a whole artichoke properly, but the reward is lots of flavor and fiber (6 grams)—as much as you'd find in a bowl of bran flakes. It's a low-calorie treat, too, depending, of course, on what stuffing or dipping sauce goes with it. On the plus side, artichokes are rich in polyphenols, the same phytochemicals found in red wine and grapes, which are believed to protect against heart disease. One phytochemical, silymarin, found in artichokes, has been shown to protect against skin cancer in animal studies. It is also a fair source of magnesium, a mineral that defends against many of the disorders of aging.

There are just 60 calories in a steamed whole artichoke, 37 in ½ cup of artichoke hearts.

Asparagus—Elegant Spears of Spring

One of the lovely signs of spring is the appearance of slender asparagus stalks in the market. Besides delectable flavor, a helping of asparagus offers lots of heart-helping potassium plus vitamin A and folate for protection against cancer. One of the important B vitamins, folate is also distinguished for the protection against birth defects it gives women in their child-bearing years. Asparagus is high in glutathione, an amino-acid combo that fights carcinogens. Dieters can dine royally on asparagus without feeling the least bit deprived of life's good things.

Enjoy 6 spears or ½ cup of sliced asparagus for only 22 calories.

Broccoli—Perhaps the Ultimate Health Machine

Even in a list of the multihealthy vegetables, broccoli is a natural leader. It's ultra-high in beta-carotene, and very rich in vitamin C. And it also delivers niacin, calcium, thiamine, phosphorus, potassium, iron, and protein. But wait, there's more! Broccoli adds needed fiber to your diet as well as the phytochemicals associated with reduced risk of cancer. Fresh broccoli, when cooked tender-crisp, has a wonderful texture, especially for salads, but frozen broccoli spears often contain even more beta-carotene (because they include more buds).

All this, and low-calorie, too: 1 cup broccoli is a mere 44 calories.

Cabbage and Brussels Sprouts—Health Builders, Great and Small

From bok choy to savoy, from red to green, cabbage in its many guises is easy to grow and tolerant of long storage, which has made it a dietary mainstay of many cultures. Current research has revealed what a great health builder this rather humble vegetable has been all along, virtues shared with its tiny replica, the brussels sprout. Both are cancer-preventing cruciferous vegetables with some especially potent phytochemicals: indoles, sulforaphane, and phenethyl isothiocyanate, a lung protector. They're chock-full of antioxidant vitamin C, too, to keep you younger longer.

There are only 16 calories in 1 cup of shredded green cabbage; 30 calories in 4 brussels sprouts.

Count on Carrots All Year Long

A vegetable to depend on in all seasons, the ubiquitous carrot is a top source of alpha carotene and beta-carotene, part of the antioxidant defense against the degeneration of aging. These two carotenes work with others to protect eyesight in later years. Also a heart protector, a "dose" of two carrots a day has been shown to substantially reduce cholesterol. Popular with cooks and dieters, carrots are second only to beets in natural sugar content. They add a touch of sweetness to stews and soups as well as making a satisfying snack food all on their own.

Crunch away! There are only 31 calories in 1 medium raw carrot.

Cauliflower—an Incredible Edible

Would you believe that one cup of cauliflower contains more vitamin C than the RDA? That alone should make cauliflower a star vegetable, since vitamin C is noted for contributing to healthy lungs and gums, wound healing, and defense against infection. As a bonus, this "cabbage with a college education" (as Mark Twain called it) is also a cruciferous cancer fighter. And cauliflower gives you potassium for your heart, boron for strong bones, and B vitamins to guard against nervous stress.

It's an all-around great vegetable at 30 calories for 1 cup of cooked cauliflower.

Celery and Fennel—Dieter's Delights

These two members of the feathery-leafed *umbelliferae* family contain phthalides, a cancer-fighting phytochemical. Since ancient times, Asians have asserted that celery lowers blood pressure, a claim that has been validated by modern research, even though this vegetable is higher than most in sodium. Two to four stalks a day have been found effective in helping to control blood pressure. Fennel, which crunches like celery but has a licorice flavor, is often (incorrectly) called "anise" in grocery markets. It's a pow-erhouse of vitamins: 1 cup of chopped fennel contains 150 percent of the RDA for vitamin C as well as large amounts of vitamin A, calcium, and potassium.

A stalk of celery contains a minuscule 6 calories; 1 cup of chopped fennel has 27.

Corn—a Fiberful American Favorite

A gift from the Native Americans, corn is a stick-to-the-ribs vegetable that is rich in carbohydrates for sustained energy and fiber for a healthy digestion. It offers some B vitamins, notably pyridoxine (vitamin B_6), a heart helper. Corn is also a source of melatonin, a hormonal substance that boosts the immune system and enhances restful sleep. A universal favorite, sweet corn is enjoyed even by those who don't care for stronger-flavored vegetables.

Corn contains 137 calories per cup, or about 70 in a 5-inch ear.

Eggplant—from the Mediterranean with Love

Eggplant's chief nutrient is folate, which has been found to protect against colorectal cancer and birth defects. This Mediterranean tempter also contains protease inhibitors, thought to suppress the malignant process for all cancers. In addition, eggplant may lower cholesterol, counteract the effect of fatty foods, and act as an antibacterial agent. Its one drawback is that eggplant absorbs more oil than any other vegetable, so it's best not to sauté the vegetable in traditional fashion. A fast stir-fry absorbs less oil, or, even better, bake or broil the slices.

Although there are only 26 calories in 1 cup of diced cooked eggplant, 5 ounces of eggplant parmigiana cooked the old-fashioned way can yield nearly 300 calories.

Garlic—Good for What Ails You

Allicin, a phytochemical found in garlic, makes this super flavor-enhancer so good for you, it ought to be prescribed as preventive medicine. Among its many claims to nutritional fame, garlic lowers blood cholesterol, protects against strokes, neutralizes carcinogens, stimulates the immune system, and has antiviral, antibacterial, and antifungal properties. There are literally hundreds of studies on the efficacy of allicin going back to World War I, when doctors used garlic to keep the wounded free of infection. It's even good for pets: A pill form of garlic and brewer's yeast is given to dogs to discourage fleas. Cooked garlic, which retains most of its preventive properties, is easiest to digest.

If you're fearful of offending with garlic breath, feed the odorous bulb to your friends and family so they won't notice. A lingering scent of garlic on the cook's hands may be deodorized with a lemon-slice scrub.

Three cloves of garlic are a bargain at 13 calories.

Greens, Dark and Leafy—Lean Nutrition Machines

If your mother urged you to "eat your greens" (as mine did), her advice was better than she knew, because it's only recently that studies have begun to show the antioxidant power and disease-preventing properties of dark, leafy vegetables. In general, greens are rich in B vitamins, vitamin C, iron, calcium, and boron for strong bones, and in the anticancer phytochemicals sulforaphane and indoles.

With slight variations, depending on the specific one, all greens are in a low-calorie range, somewhere between 11 calories per ½ cup for cooked mustard greens and 21 for the same amount of spinach.

Mushrooms: Magic for the Immune System

Because they lack the bright colors of many vegetables—no chlorophyll and therefore no beta-carotene or vitamin C—mushrooms were not regarded as nutritious. Now we know, however, they're a good source of B vitamins, potassium, chromium, and copper. Mushrooms build immunity, especially the shiitake, which contains lentinan, an antiviral substance. In recent tests in Japan, this potent mushroom has shown promising results as a flu drug, and Japanese researchers claim the shiitake has proved to be more effective than AZT against AIDS.

Cautions: It's best to cook mushrooms; raw mushrooms contain hydrazines, tumor-producing substances that are lost in cooking. And never, never pick mushrooms in the wild; there are many deadly varieties out there!

There are only 21 calories in a cup of cooked (steamed, not fried) mushrooms.

Onions, Leeks, Scallions, Shallots, and Chives

Sharing many of the healthful properties of garlic, these flavor enliveners, mainstays of soups, stews, and sautés in every country's cuisine, are good preventive medicine for the heart: They lower the damaging LDL cholesterol, raise the helpful HDL cholesterol (page 26), and help to keep the blood from clotting, thus preventing strokes. Populations whose cuisines are rich in onions seem less at risk for stomach cancer as well. Onions and their bulbous family are infection fighters, too, so keep chopping them into salads during cold and flu season.

These figures won't make you cry: 30 calories in ½ cup of raw onions, 16 calories in the same amount of cooked leeks.

Peppers and Chiles—Zing for Your Diet

It sometimes comes as a surprise that green bell peppers contain twice as much antioxidant vitamin C as oranges. But that's not all—red bell peppers contain three times as much, and hot chiles even more! Red bells are also a great source of beta-carotene. Pungent chiles find their claim to healthy fame in capsaicin, the "hot stuff" that's linked to cardiovascular health. The whole respiratory system "breathes easier" with capsaicin, which opens air passages, acting as an expectorant and a decongestant, so when you have a cold, try a dash of hot pepper sauce in your bowl of chicken soup. Another surprise—that fiery capsaicin

doesn't burn your stomach; it actually helps to prevent ulcers.

Some scientists theorize that hot-chile lovers experience a "high" from endorphins—substances released by the brain in response to discomfort—similar to a "runner's high."

Caution: Handling hot chiles can cause an allergic reaction. Wear rubber gloves when preparing them; don't touch your eyes; and don't inhale their fumes. The hottest parts of hot chiles are the ribs and seeds.

Lots of zing for only 17 calories in ½ cup of chopped hot chiles; 13 calories if you opt for sweet bell peppers instead.

Potatoes, White and Sweet— Terrific Tubers

Sweet potatoes offer such a bonanza of beta-carotene that they hardly need any other virtue to be labeled super. Although we call the orangey potatoes "yams," they're really a moister variety of sweet potatoes; true yams are grown only in the tropics. Even without all that glorious carotene, white potatoes are a very nutritious vegetable, with B vitamins, chromium, and cancer-fighting protease inhibitors. White or sweet, both are carbohydrate foods that calm the mind and sustain the body during strenuous physical activity. All potatoes are chock-full of potassium for a healthy heart and are good sources of vitamin C as well.

Caution: Although white potato skins are rich in fiber, iron, and chromium, peel off and discard any green patches and sprouts, which develop when white potato skins are exposed to light. These may harbor solanine, a somewhat toxic chemical that can cause diarrhea and headache.

Although so much sweeter, a 5-inch sweet potato has 120 calories compared to 145 in a slightly smaller white potato. A fine diet food if no fat is added, so try a topping of nonfat plain yogurt and chopped chives.

Squashes (summer)—Prolific in Potassium
Another great diet food to fill up on, summer squashes—from yellow straight or crookneck to green zucchini—are 95 percent water. Not great vitamin sources, and yet these easily grown, abundant summer favorites are rich in potassium to combat high blood pressure and strokes. Because they are consumed with shell and seeds, they give us a good serving of fiber for a healthy digestive system. Unlike eggplant, with which they are often teamed, zucchini don't act like sponges when they are sautéed; instead they become very flavorful while leaving most of the oil still in the skillet.

Just 18 calories in ½ cup of summer squash slices, 14 in zucchini. Indulge!

Squash (winter) and Pumpkin—Plump with Beta-carotene
As American as apple pie, all squashes are gourds native to our continent. These orange-fleshed, long-keeping winter staples, which once nourished Native Americans and early European settlers, still offer us many health benefits for which to give thanks. They are rich in antioxidant beta-carotene, converted by our bodies into cold-fighting vitamin A. The carotenes are high on the list of anticancer foods as well as enhancers of the immune system, and therefore protective against bacteria and viruses. Sweet, dense, yet virtually fat-free, these vegetables offer plenty of sustaining complex carbohydrates as well. Pumpkin is a fine source of heart-helping potassium.

They're all low in calories, with variations according to kind. One-half cup cooked Hubbard squash has 51 calories; butternut, 41; spaghetti, only 23. One-half cup cooked pumpkin yields 24 calories.

Tomatoes—a Versatile Favorite Full of Hidden Virtues
Although native to the Americas, tomatoes didn't find their claim to fame until some inspired Spanish chef sautéed them with peppers, garlic, and oil, thus making culinary history. It's been estimated that tomatoes have over ten thousand phytochemicals, so we've only just begun to learn all there is to know about this vegetable's virtues. Tomatoes are an excellent source of lycopene, the carotenoid that defends against prostate as well as other forms of cancer, and are a major source of antiaging, antistress melatonin. As an antioxidant–vitamin C vegetable, tomatoes work diligently at cleaning up free radicals, those troublemakers that cause cell damage and the diseases of aging. Even people

who aren't great vegetable lovers seem to find tomatoes tempting and tasty—another bonus to the cook. (If all else fails, nap it with tomato sauce!)

Your average raw tomato weighs in at 26 calories; 1 cup of stewed tomatoes is 80 calories.

Turnips and Rutabagas—Root for Root Vegetables!

As so often happens with foods associated with poor farmers, these two terrific vegetables are rich in health benefits. As part of the cruciferous family, they're especially high in anticancer phytochemicals. Turnips are white-fleshed; rutabagas (a kind of turnip-cabbage) are yellow-fleshed and therefore also a source of antioxidant beta-carotene as well as vitamin C. Not bad for peasant food! The longer you cook turnips or rutabagas, the stronger their flavor—something to keep in mind if you like your vegetables mild. Tiny white turnips are lovely sliced raw, like radishes, into a salad.

Rutabagas are 29 calories for ½ cup; turnips 14 calories—so have a guilt-free second helping!

The Anti-Aging Fruits

Look younger and stay healthier with fabulous fruits, nature's really-good-for-you desserts. They're so delectable that you'd never guess they're rich in nutrients and chemicals to ward off the effects of aging.

Population diet research has turned up the good news that people who eat more fruits and vegetables simply live longer and healthier lives. Some special attention should be paid to the orange-fleshed fruits such as papaya and nectarines for their abundant beta-carotene content. Science now believes that beta-carotene *plus the phytochemicals with which it naturally combines* defends the body against many cancers.

Another great group, the citrus fruits, is notable for a variety of phytochemicals as well as for plentiful vitamin C—a combination that protects against cancer at all stages.

As sources of vitamin A and C, citrus and orange-fleshed fruits play an important role, too, in nourishing the skin, which becomes thinner and dryer with advancing years. What you put on your skin may help keep its moisture from evaporating, but it's what you eat that really nurtures the body's outer layer. The high water content of fruits is also important (as is drinking lots of water) in keeping skin hydrated and supple. Some fruits are 90 percent water, and yet so filled with good nutrition in that other 10 percent!

Apples—Super Snack for Busy People
An apple a day . . . Actually it's two or three apples a day that have been found in one study to be the prescription for lowering blood cholesterol 10 percent or more—an effect credited to their high content of pectin, a soluble fiber. But as with all whole foods, there may be other factors as yet undiscovered, since the actual apple is

more effective than isolated supplementary pectin—and more fun to eat, too. Apples are high in another heart saver, potassium, and in boron, a trace mineral that helps to prevent bone loss. Apples and apple juice fight bacteria and viruses, including the cold virus, and are anti-inflammatory. Known as "nature's toothbrush," raw apples have tooth-cleaning and gum-stimulating properties that make them a perfect dessert for the brown-bag set (who may not be able to brush after lunch).

A medium raw apple eaten with its skin is 81 calories, so munch away!

Apricots—Sweets Can Be Super, Too!

If someone at your house won't eat carrots and squash, feed them apricots! The same abundant beta-carotene goodness of orange vegetables is also present in the orange fruits. Naturally high in vitamin A and potassium, apricots are also a great source of vitamin C and natural fiber. And they're higher in phosphorus and calcium than most other fruits.

Caution: The seed of an apricot kernel is poisonous if eaten in quantity; it's the source of laetrile.

Three raw apricots have 51 calories. Even apricots in heavy syrup—hardly a health food—can be indulged in for only 75 calories in four halves. And if you snack on ten dried apricot halves, you'll consume 83 calories and almost enough vitamin A to qualify as a supplement.

Avocados—Fatty but Fine Fruit

Although avocados have a high fat content, it's a monounsaturated fat (like olive oil) that actually helps to lower blood cholesterol. This deep green, pear-shaped fruit is high in potassium, making it an anti-stroke food. Avocados are a great source of glutathione, which has been found to block thirty carcinogens. Composed of amino acids, glutathione is manufactured by the body to detoxify potentially dangerous substances; it's also found in some foods, with avocados at the head of the list. High in folate, a B-vitamin cancer fighter, an avocado is a fruit of many virtues.

Half of a medium avocado from California is 153 calories; the Florida variety is 170.

Bananas—Heart-Smart and Stomach Soothing

Bananas are great as a breakfast food (especially for those who are afflicted with a "nervy tummy" in the morning) or for a late-night snack, and here's why. As a stomach soother, substances in banana powder have proved effective in lessening ulcer activity in animal tests. As a complex-carbohydrate food, bananas share in the carbo-calming effect. And bananas are a two-way natural source of melatonin, a sleep-inducing and stress-relieving hormone: first, because they're high on the list of foods that contain melatonin itself, and second, because they're rich in vitamin B_6 (as is the so-called "cooking banana," the plantain), which stimulates melatonin production in the body. The older you get, the more liable you are to be deficient in vitamin B$_6$, just when you need melatonin most.

More benefits: Bananas are also high in potassium and magnesium—both heart protectors. All this, and a banana comes in its own neat easily opened package! Bananas belong in every fruit bowl. If the last few in a bunch threaten to overripen, put them in a white plastic bag in the refrigerator for longer keeping.

A medium banana contains 105 calories, but only a trace of fat.

Berries—"Good Things Come in Small Packages"

All berries are super sources of ellagic acid, which may help to prevent certain kinds of cancer. Although sweet and delicate, berries promote a healthy digestive tract with their high fiber content. Cranberries and blueberries have been shown to contain compounds that prevent microbes from adhering to the bladder wall and triggering a urinary tract infection. According to medical folklore, blueberries help to cure diarrhea, perhaps because blueberries as well as black currants are high in anthocyanosides, substances that fight infectious bacteria, including *E. coli*. Raspberries are antioxidant, antiviral, and contain an aspirinlike compound. Strawberries are high in potassium for heart health and vitamin C for keeping free radicals in check. In population-diet studies, people who ate the most strawberries developed fewer cancers. Although this type of research

doesn't prove cause and effect, it does provide indications of what constitutes a healthy diet. And berries belong!

Berries are generally low in calories: per cup, blueberries, 82 calories; raspberries, 61 calories; and strawberries, a mere 45 calories.

Citrus Fruits—a Bonanza of Cancer Fighters

We've all learned that citrus fruits are a top source of vitamin C and beta-carotene, a dynamic duo for cleaning up the free radicals that accelerate disorders associated with aging. But it's less well known that this cornucopia of oranges, grapefruit, tangerines, lemons, and limes contains the greatest package of specific cancer-fighting phytochemicals that have been found in any food—over fifty of them, and still counting! Some scientists theorize that a mixture of phytochemicals works more powerfully together in whole foods than they do as separate supplements. Among these, one of the most potent flavonoids in inhibiting the invasiveness of cancer, tangeretin, has been found in tangerines.

Grapefruit contains a unique cholesterol-lowering cocktail not found in other citrus. It's found in the membranes, so you have to eat the whole grapefruit, not just drink the juice, in order to reap this additional benefit.

A medium orange has 65 calories; a tangerine, 37 calories; and a half grapefruit, 39. A chilled juicy tangerine makes a great snack while watching television.

Figs—Honeyed Goodness, Fresh or Dried

Black Mission, Calimyrna, Dakota, and Brown Turkey figs—even the names are lush and exotic! That supple skin encloses a host of sweet, edible seeds responsible for the high insoluble fiber content of figs. They also contain pectin, which offers soluble fiber as well. Figs are also a good source of the minerals potassium (for the heart), iron (for energy), and zinc (for immunity). Medical folklore claimed figs to be a treatment for cancer; in modern research, a substance found in figs, benzaldehyde, is being studied for its ability to shrink tumors in laboratory animals. Besides their antitumor properties, figs are antibacterial and antiparasitic. So if you're craving a chewy sweet treat, stick with figs instead of candy.

Five dried figs are 27 calories; one medium fresh fig is 37.

Grapes—the Great Snack Food

Although their vitamin content is negligible, grapes are outstanding snacks in other ways. All grapes are rich in boron, which helps prevent the bone loss of advancing years; chromium, a blood sugar regulator; and cancer-fighting polyphenols. Red grapes (and the wine made from them) contain an extra couple of phytochemicals, resveratrol and quercetin, that inhibit blood clotting, lower the damaging LDL cholesterol, and raise the helpful HDL cholesterol. Adding to the heart-saving profile of grapes, raisins made from them are high in potassium and fiber. Resveratrol and quercetin have been credited with saving the wine-loving French from the effects of their high-fat diet. Although this is a somewhat controversial claim in nutrition circles, because excessive alcohol is definitely detrimental to health, if you do enjoy a glass of red wine with dinner, it may be doing your heart good, too.

In the most recent animal research, resveratrol, found in the skins of red grapes, was also shown to stop the development of cancer at any of three different stages. Scientists are now trying to isolate resveratrol to test it as a cancer medicine.

A cup of grapes contains only 58 calories, but there are 150 calories in 1/3 cup of raisins. But raisins used sparingly as a flavoring agent in desserts, cookies, and sweet breads are a healthy choice compared to, say, chocolate chips.

Kiwifruit—Supreme for Vitamin C

It's known as the Chinese gooseberry, but it's named for a New Zealand bird and looks like a large fuzzy brown egg. Its bright green interior and design of edible black seeds have made it popular as a garnish. Yet the kiwi's claim to fruit fame should be its amazing vitamin C content. When you eat a single kiwi, you're consuming one and a half times your RDA of vitamin C. (But considering all the health benefits of vitamin C, the RDA might be considered only the starting place.) A kiwi is also an excellent source of potassium for the heart and fiber for the digestive tract.

Kiwis contain a meat-tenderizing enzyme called actinidin. As a tenderizer, the fruit can be crushed and used in a marinade or simply rubbed over both sides of a piece of meat a half hour before grilling. But don't put kiwi in a gelatin; actinidin will prevent it from setting.

Indulge in a whole medium kiwi for only 46 calories.

Mango—a Tropical Treat That's Big on Beta-carotene

Whenever you eat an orange-fleshed fruit or vegetable, you can count on getting lots of vitamin A from carotenoids, and mangoes are a perfect example. It's particularly high in beta cryptoxanthin, a lesser-known carotenoid that fights lung cancer. But the antiaging antioxidant power of mangoes doesn't end there; they're also rich in vitamin C and contain a respectable amount of vitamin E as well (a rarity among fruits). Mangoes are big on potassium, helping to control blood pressure, too. Although a bit messy to peel and pit, their goodness and delectable flavor make them well worth the effort.

Treat yourself to half a medium mango for just 68 calories.

Melons—Super Summer Favorites

It may seem that watermelon is little more than cool, sweetened water in fruit form, but actually this big picnic favorite is one of the best sources of lycopene and glutathione, two super cancer fighters. Watermelon is antibacterial as well.

Orange-fleshed cantaloupe is a powerhouse of vitamins A and C. Cantaloupe, honeydew, and watermelon are good sources of heart-helping potassium.

High water content means low in calories, so you can feast on diced melon for somewhere between 50 and 60 calories a cup.

Papaya—Tenderizer of the Tropics

Papaya is the source of papain, the chief ingredient in meat tenderizers sold in the supermarket. In tropical countries, cooks often wrap meat in papaya leaves or use chunks of the unripe fruit as a tenderizing marinade (ripe papaya doesn't contain as much papain). Because papain breaks down protein, it's also used in natural digestion aids sold by health food stores.

High in vitamin C and in vitamin A, papaya is as good for you as it is luscious. Like the mango, it contains beta cryptoxanthin, a carotenoid that defends against lung cancer. A high pectin content makes papaya a cholesterol-lowering fruit, and it also provides a helping of folate to decrease the risk of clogged arteries.

A medium papaya contains 117 calories—share it with a friend for 59 calories each.

Peaches and Nectarines—You'd Never Guess They're Health Food

They're not all Georgia peaches anymore—California, Washington, South Carolina, and several other states have got into the act, growing hundreds of varieties of cling and freestone fruit, both fuzzy peaches and smooth-skinned, honeyed nectarines. The two fruits are great sources of vitamin A and potassium, and fair sources of vitamin C. They're high on the glutathione list, too, placing them among the cancer-deterrent fruits, and they contain boron for bone strength. In recipes, you'll find peaches and nectarines are handily interchangeable with each other and with fresh apricots.

Thirty-seven calories in a medium peach—better have two! Nectarines, on the other hand, are somewhat sweeter and denser, at 67 calories.

Pineapple—a Powerful Medicine for Bones

Named for its resemblance to a pinecone, pineapples are a sweet-tart fruit of many health benefits. For openers, they're anti-inflammatory, antiviral, antibacterial, and help to dissolve blood clots. Like many fruits, pineapples are high in wound-healing vitamin C. But unlike the others, they're also a top source of manganese, which enhances bone metabolism and helps to prevent osteoporosis. Making pineapple juice one of your juice drinks helps to ward off this crippling disorder.

Pineapple contains the enzyme bromelain, which may account for many of its healing properties. Since bromelain digests protein, that makes pineapple a digestive aid. (Sometimes as we age, indigestion comes from lack of sufficient gastric juices, including hydrochloric acid, to break down protein—*atrophic gastritis*—rather

than from too much acid.) This enzymatic action also allows pineapple to qualify as a great meat tenderizer, but it's recommended that meat not be left in a pineapple marinade for longer than 10 minutes! Because of bromelain, raw pineapple will keep a gelatin mixture from setting, but canned pineapple, which has been "cooked," is okay for use.

A cup of raw pineapple has 77 calories; or 150 calories for canned pineapple in juice pack.

Prunes and Dates—Instant Energy

They have a concentrated sweetness that's high in calories, it's true, but prunes and dates have health benefits that make them much better choices for an instant energy buzz than, say, a candy bar. Both treats are high in potassium, fiber, and vitamin B_6, all heart helpers, and in iron, for energy that goes beyond that quick sugar boost. Some studies have indicated that dates may protect against pancreatic cancer. Their high boron content helps to prevent calcium loss in bones.

Prunes are a source of natural aspirin. They're also mightily laxative, but the USDA, after years of research, has given up trying to find out why prunes and prune juice have this effect. It could be prunes' high magnesium content, fiber, or sorbitol, a natural sugar, but other dried fruits with some of these same substances are not laxative. The conclusion is that it's the particular combination of nutrients and nonnutrients with perhaps some unknown

elements that makes prunes relieve constipation. Although we don't know the cause
yet, their effect has been well proven.

Snacking on five dates will add 114 calories to your daily fare; five prunes contain
100 calories.

The Anti-Aging Grains, Legumes, Nuts, and Seeds

Grains and legumes are an outstanding
source of fiber, both soluble and insoluble.
Soluble fiber lowers cholesterol and insoluble fiber protects against various disorders
and diseases of the colon.

Vitamin E is also abundant in this food
group (and in oils). Of all the antioxidant
vitamins, this one may be the most difficult
to find in food sources at levels sufficient to
be meaningful. This is especially true for
dieters who will naturally be avoiding oils
and high-calorie foods like nuts. But since
vitamin E is a great heart protector, it's well
worth making the effort to add more
whole grains, beans, and peas to your daily
fare.

At the base of the food pyramid, grains,
pasta, and rice are also rich in cancer-fighting phytochemicals, such as protease
inhibitors, and in B vitamins that nourish
the whole nervous system and build brain
power, among many other benefits.

A margarine called Benecol® being mar-
keted in Finland has been shown to lower
cholesterol. Two tablespoons a day of this
"foodaceutical" have reduced mildly ele-
vated cholesterol by 10 percent or more.

The active ingredient is sitostanol, an
extract of pine oil, also found in nuts and
grains.

Both beans and grains are rich in protein, but it's an incomplete protein. When
combined, however, in dishes like black
beans and rice or tortillas with vegetable
chili or even a peanut butter sandwich on
whole-wheat bread, each makes up for
what the other lacks in amino acids,
thereby completing the protein profile. So
beans and grains when eaten together provide high-quality protein and are a perfectly good meat substitute.

Also important to vegetarians, grains
and legumes are good sources of vegetable
iron (non-heme), which fights ordinary
fatigue as well as anemia. Iron ferries oxygen around the body, so to think clearly
and feel energetic, vegetarians need the
iron that foods like grains and beans provide.

Whole grains and brown rice are rich in
pyridoxine, vitamin B_6, which is credited
with keeping homocysteine in check. If the
amino acid homocysteine builds up in the
system, it injures blood vessels; high levels
are considered a warning of future heart
attacks. Good bread made from unrefined
grains is a true "staff of life" that keeps the
cardiovascular system healthy.

Barley—a Neglected Heart Saver

It's rather an overlooked food in this country, and yet barley is right up there with
oats as a cholesterol-lowering grain that
ought to be part of the diets of all health-

oriented people. Pearled barley, with the bran removed, is the most widely available form of this great grain. Pot barley, also called Scotch barley, still contains part of the bran layer (and therefore more of the B-vitamin content) and is worth seeking out at health food stores.

Barley is credited with being antiviral and anticarcinogenic, with a good helping of cancer-fighting folate in every dishful.

A cup of cooked barley contains 193 calories. Try it as a replacement for rice in a pilaf or a salad.

Beans—Humble and Healthy

You can't get better nutrition for your food dollar than this humble health food provides. Beans are a good source of potassium and fiber for a healthy heart. Besides lowering cholesterol, beans also help to regulate blood sugar, making them a good food for diabetics. Other nutrients in beans include boron and manganese for keeping bones strong in later life, iron for energy, zinc for building immunity, thiamine for memory, and protease inhibitors for protecting against cancer. What a bargain!

Green beans share in all the benefits of dried beans, but to a lesser degree, since they're not as dense. On the plus side, they're a good source of vitamins A and C, which dried beans lack. Green beans are also much lower in calorie count.

Soybeans deserve some special notice all on their own. Of all the plant foods, soybeans come nearest to being a complete protein. Besides sharing all the other health benefits of beans, this Asian staple is richly endowed with chemical compounds that help the body to block cancer growth at every stage. New research suggests that high soy consumption may be a major factor in Japan's low breast cancer incidence. Soy is rich in phytoestrogens, plant estrogens that suppress the damaging effects of hormonal estrogen, thought to be implicated in breast cancer. Plant estrogens also have been shown to minimize menopausal symptoms by making up for the body's diminishing supply. Soy protein sprinkled on cereal, for instance, made hot flashes more bearable in one study, and was responsible for lowering cholesterol and blood pressure. Soybeans also contain a supply of choline, a memory booster. They may prevent or dissolve gallstones, as they have been shown to dissolve kidney stones in animals. A chameleon food of many forms, soybeans can be enjoyed as tofu, miso, tempeh, soy nuts, soy milk, soy flour, or the beans themselves.

For bean counters, 1 cup of pea (navy) beans has 224 calories; kidney beans, 218; limas, 189, lentils, 231; green beans, 31; soybeans, 234. Tofu (firm) has 183 calories per 1/2 cup. Before you gasp over the high figures, compare them to a 3.5-ounce broiled beef patty at 289 calories—and that's a small patty.

Cornmeal, the Pilgrims' Mainstay

As a refined grain, the cornmeal you find in supermarkets doesn't offer all the corn goodness of whole cornmeal (sometimes called "unbolted cornmeal"), which still contains the bran and germ. Look for whole cornmeal in natural foods stores; it is usually stone ground. Polenta, on which the Italian dish of the same name is based, is a coarsely ground cornmeal, and either refined or whole cornmeal, if coarse, can be used to make it. In any case, all cornmeal provides a healthy helping of potassium and phosphorus, which are good not only for the heart but also for mental alertness. These two minerals combine to send oxygen to the brain and, with calcium, to regulate neuromuscular activity. Cornmeal is also a good source of vitamin A and has antiviral and anticancer properties. Whole cornmeal adds more fiber and more B vitamins.

A half cup of whole cornmeal has 221 calories. If it is in the form of homemade corn bread, one piece will contain 172 calories. A cup of cooked cornmeal or polenta is 120 calories.

Flaxseed—a Powerhouse of Prevention

The new darling of the health food circuit is more than just trendy; flaxseed really lives up to the translation of its Latin name (*Linum usitatissimum*) "most useful." It's been extensively studied and endorsed by the FDA, whose research has shown that flaxseed stimulates the immune system and lowers total cholesterol as well as improves the ratio between "good" HDL and "bad" LDL blood cholesterol. It's the richest natural source of the omega-3 essential fatty acids. The only other substantial sources of omega-3s are seafood and walnuts, so if you're not a fish lover, flaxseed is a good substitute. Americans, while consuming perhaps more of the omega-6 fatty acids (found in meats) than they need, as a rule are *not* getting all the omega-3s they could use to ward off heart disease, inflammatory ailments like rheumatism, and other illnesses that come with age.

Flaxseed contains all nine essential amino acids, more potassium per serving than a banana, plus it's loaded with lignans, phytochemicals that are linked to low incidence of breast and colon cancer. Milled flaxseed can be added to baked goods, such as breads and pizzas, imparting a rather nutty new flavor. You can find cracked flaxseed and milled flaxseed in natural foods stores and some catalogs, such as the King Arthur Flour Baker's Catalog.

In 1 tablespoon of milled flaxseed there are about 70 calories.

Nuts and Seeds Are High-Energy Foods

No wonder little woodland creatures pack away nuts for the winter; they couldn't find a more concentrated kind of nutrition than the formula nature puts into its seed foods. In general, nuts contain boron and magnesium to build bones, iron to build blood, choline to enhance memory, niacin to protect the heart, and fiber to keep the digestive tract healthy. They're among the best plant sources of protein.

Walnuts supply those elusive omega-3

fatty acids usually only found in fish and flaxseed, plus lots of antioxidant vitamin E. Almonds are also rich in vitamin E, and they're a surprising source of calcium as well. Cashews and peanuts (and their butters!) are big on folate. Chestnuts are the lowest in fat of all the nuts (macadamias are the highest). Brazil nuts have a unique claim to nutritional fame: They're such an amazing source of selenium that it's best to snack on them moderately—two a day is plenty.

Sunflower, sesame, and pumpkin seeds are equally packed with nutrition. They're high in protein and are good sources of the B-vitamin complex as well as vitamins A, D, and E. Pumpkin and squash seeds are high in iron; sesame, in calcium; and sunflower, in calcium, potassium, and phosphorus.

The seasoning seeds have important properties, too, in the annals of herbal medicine. Fennel, anise, and caraway are digestive aids; celery seed is a diuretic and a sedative.

With the exception of coconut, the oils in nuts and seeds are unsaturated, so although they're high in fat and calories, they're still good for you, in moderation.

An ounce of walnuts (14 halves) contains 182 calories; cashews, 163; almonds, 166; Brazil nuts, 186; peanuts, 170. Pumpkin and squash seeds contain 154 calories per ounce (but that's 142 seeds!); sunflower seeds, 162 calories. Sesame seeds have 47 calories per tablespoon.

Oats—Health Secret of the Robust Scots

Lucky for us, oats are one grain that's not automatically refined by the producers. With its bran intact, a breakfast dish of oatmeal still offers us a wealth of whole-grain goodness. For openers, oats are high in the soluble fiber beta glucan, which is responsible for meaningful reduction in cholesterol for those who eat as little as a cup of cooked oatmeal every day—or two ounces dry, if you'd prefer to add your oats to muffins, breads, meat loaf, and the like. Even the cautious FDA is allowing a leading manufacturer of oatmeal to advertise its heart healthfulness on the label.

But that's only the beginning. Oats are rich in complex carbohydrates, and they supply vitamin E, folate, protein, iron, manganese, copper, and zinc as well. They're also one of the best food sources of melatonin, which has recently come to the attention of the health-conscious. Melatonin is a powerful antioxidant that's credited with inducing restful sleep, relieving jet lag, and stimulating the immune system. The body manufactures its own melatonin, but since its production can slow down with age, a helping of oats may fill in nicely. In addition, a psychoactive compound in oats is thought to help relieve depression. With all of this to recommend oats, it's a shame that most of the world's crop is fed to animals. In Scotland, however, they really know their oats, and Scottish cookbooks abound in ways to use this impressive grain.

There are 159 calories in 1 cup of

cooked oatmeal, and you can't find a finer start to a cold winter's morning.

Peas—Great Vegetable Protein!

Nature intended peas to nourish new plants, so they're packed with energy. Of all the vegetables, only fresh limas are higher in protein than green peas: A scant cup has more (but incomplete) protein than a whole egg, but with hardly any fat. Snow peas have less protein but are rich in calcium. All peas are a good source of complex carbohydrates, B-complex vitamins to nourish the nervous system, and antioxidant vitamins A and C. Alas, the season for fresh peas is extremely short, but frozen (not canned) peas are a good substitute during the rest of the year.

A cup of cooked peas contains 114 calories—and lots of pizzazz!

Quinoa—an Old Grain Is Rediscovered

Ancient staple of the Incas, quinoa (pronounced *keen*-wa) has come to life again on the shelves of natural food stores because of its great food value. Although quinoa has been called a "supergrain," it's not really a grain but a relative of Swiss chard and spinach. It cooks and looks like a grain, however, plumping up in cooking liquid to three to four times its size. Unlike "real" grains, quinoa contains a high-quality, complete protein, which is its chief claim to nutritional fame and what makes it an excellent food for vegetarians. But more than protein, quinoa is also a great source of iron, magnesium, potassium, phosphorus, zinc, and several B vitamins. Definitely worth trying, quinoa can be substituted for rice as a complement for stews.

Note: Quinoa should be rinsed before cooking. Nature provided quinoa with a bitter coating (saponin) to protect it from insects. The quinoa sold in this country has been processed to remove this coating; rinsing simply ensures that no traces remain to spoil the nutty flavor.

A half cup of uncooked quinoa contains 318 calories, but remember that the grains will increase greatly in volume when cooked.

Rice—Brown, White, and Wild

The staple food of more than half the world, rice is the least allergenic of grains. A cereal made from rice is often one of the first solid foods fed to babies. Easily digested and antidiarrheal, rice's mild goodness is a complex-carbohydrate comforter at all ages. Because it contains protease inhibitors, it's an anticancer food as well. White rice loses its vitamins and minerals in the refining process; so-called "enriched" rice returns some of them, but to enjoy the full value of the B vitamins, magnesium, phosphorus, and heart-helping soluble fiber that should be there, choose brown rice. Brown rice does take longer to cook, so make more than is needed for one meal and enjoy it for several days. Among its other virtues, rice is high on the list of foods that contain melatonin, a strong antioxidant defender against the aging process.

Wild rice is a great food, too, although it's not really rice, botanically speaking, but the seed of an aquatic grass. It contains twice the protein of regular rice and is especially rich in folate and zinc.

A cup of white long-grain rice is 264 calories; 1 cup of brown long-grain is less, 216; and wild rice, only 166.

Wheat Germ—Heart of the Wheat

The oldest of grains, its origins lost in antiquity, wheat has been the staff of life in European cuisines for countless generations. Unfortunately, in an effort to refine wheat and its products, this grain often is milled to eliminate the bran and germ, resulting in delicate white flour lacking its most nutritious parts. Enriched white flour puts back some of the lost B vitamins but not the important fiber content that the bran provides.

So many important vitamins and vital minerals are contained in whole wheat and wheat germ that it qualifies as one of the stars of antiaging. To begin with, it offers nearly all the B vitamins for a healthy nervous system, as well as choline, chromium, copper, magnesium, manganese, potassium, and zinc. In this long list are the nutrients that help to keep the heart, metabolic system, and memory in top form. Wheat germ is also a great source of that dynamic duo, vitamin E and selenium, which build immunity to the diseases of aging. Wheat products are complex carbohydrates, which sustain energy, and the fiber in wheat bran keeps the digestive system fit. It seems that every part of the body needs whole wheat to stay in good working order.

The prescription, then, is to choose more whole-grain breads and cereals and to cook with more whole-wheat flour. But there are even more ways to take advantage of the benefits of wheat. Plain toasted wheat germ, sold in the cereal section of supermarkets, can be easily added to breaded foods, meat loaves, and many other dishes. It adds a nutty flavor as well as super nutrition. Wheat berries, usually found in natural foods stores, are whole-wheat kernels that are boiled until soft, after which they can be introduced into soups, stews, salads, and rice dishes for extra wheat goodness.

Because of the oil it contains, 2 tablespoons of toasted wheat germ has 50 calories (10 calories of which are from fat) but no cholesterol. Be reminded that the same amount of wheat germ also contains 15 percent of your RDA for hard-to-get vitamin E plus many other goodies. A slice of whole-wheat bread contains from 60 to 80 calories, depending on brand. A cup of Wheaties® cereal is 100 calories.

The Anti-Aging Oils

Although it's fashionable these days to seek out fat-free products (while ignoring high calorie content or percentage of sugar in all those heavily advertised fat-free desserts), there is something to be said for the goodness of oils and their importance in one's diet. It's vital to reduce dietary fat, of course, but *cutting down* does not mean *cutting out*. Fats (also called lipids) have an important role to play in maintaining tissues, organs, and cells. The average adult needs 4 teaspoons of essential oils per day. Menopausal women who are suffering from dry hair, skin, and vaginal tissues may find relief in consuming even more, 2 to 3 tablespoons. Rather than becoming fat-phobic, it's better to learn which fats are actually healthful and may be considered a vital part of the anti-aging regime—and to save your "fat allowance" for the good stuff.

Some of the oils listed below are rich in the same heart-saving omega-3 fatty acids that fish contain. The omega-3s protect the heart; help to avert arthritis, cancer, and cataracts; and keep the skin youthful and healthy. Both the omega-3s and the omega-6s feed your brain and nervous system the special nutrients they need—linoleic acid and alpha-linolenic acid. The omega-6s are responsible for the transport and breakdown of blood cholesterol.

Monounsaturated oils, like olive and canola oils, lower the harmful LDL cholesterol levels while leaving the helpful HDL cholesterol unchanged. Polyunsaturated oils (corn oil, soybean, sunflower) lower both, which is not as advantageous. Simply measuring total cholesterol can be misleading. What makes the cholesterol in your blood damaging or helpful depends on the kind of fat-protein molecules that transport the cholesterol. Low-density lipoproteins (the "bad" LDL) carry cholesterol toward the coronary arteries, and high-density lipoproteins (the "good" HDL) carry cholesterol away. If your HDL level is high, the risk factors associated with LDL cholesterol are lowered. The ratio between "good" HDL and the "bad" LDL cholesterol may be more important than the bottom-line total figure.

Recently, a diet including the monounsaturated oils has been found to lower glucose levels as well as harmful LDL cholesterol in people with Type II diabetes (adult-onset diabetes).

The phrase *low cholesterol* that appears on the labels of vegetable oils, however, is meaningless. Only animal products contain cholesterol. Nevertheless, while containing no cholesterol, oils are still 100 percent fat, high in calories, and must be used judiciously. No more than 30 percent of one's daily calories ought to come from fat. Since fat is high in calories, a tablespoon of oil is the calorie equivalent of, say, 3 cups of strawberries.

The protective antioxidant vitamin that's most difficult to obtain in effective quantities is vitamin E, which is found in its most concentrated form in vegetable oils, especially olive and flaxseed. If you're not taking vitamin E in supplement form (as some physicians are now recommending), you need to be especially careful to choose vegetable oils for your "fat allotment," as well as opting for vitamin E–rich whole-grain foods.

In cooking, fats frequently enhance and carry the flavor. Just a tablespoon or so can make quite a difference to an entire dish. Onions and garlic sautéed in oil, for instance, are much more savory than if simply steamed—and much subtler and more digestible than if they were added raw to the dish.

The vegetable oils in this section contain about 120 calories and 14 grams of fat per tablespoon.

Canola Oil—a Vegetable Oil with Many Pluses

Also known as rapeseed oil, canola oil is a good source of omega-3 fatty acids for protection against heart disease and arthritis. It's also a source of omega-6s, thus providing a balance of essential fatty acids considered by nutritionists to be particularly desirable. Next to olive oil, canola is the most monounsaturated at 62 percent. Monounsaturated oils are credited with helping to lower cholesterol.

Canola oil is bland in flavor, making it a good choice as a replacement for butter in baked goods. It's also fine for stir-fries and other dishes that do not require the robust Mediterranean flavor of olive oil.

Flaxseed Oil—Especially for Those Who Aren't Fish Lovers

It's difficult to get enough of the heart-healthy omega-3 fatty acids if you don't eat fish. But flaxseed oil (and flaxseed in other forms, such as cracked or milled flaxseed) is an excellent vegetable source of the omega-3s. Its health benefits include lowering cholesterol, protecting against stroke, and slowing the progress of rheumatoid arthritis and atherosclerosis. And flaxseed oil offers a bonus to women: It contains substantial amounts of phytoestrogen (plant estrogen) lignans, which help suppress hormone-related disorders ranging from hot flashes to fibroid tumors to breast and ovarian cancer. Lignans also appear to lower the risk of colon cancer. As a bonus, adding flaxseed oil to the diet is recommended as a means of keeping aging skin supple and fresh-looking.

Available chiefly in natural foods stores, flaxseed oil should be refrigerated after opening. One way of including flaxseed oil in one's meals is to make it part of a salad oil blend, and a salad a day is always a smart move toward better nutrition.

Olive Oil—"Liquid Gold" of the Mediterranean

How a population could consume so much fat in the form of olive oil and still enjoy a reduced risk of heart disease was the question that first attracted the attention of nutrition researchers to the Mediterranean diet. It's wasn't just the oil that was responsible, of course; it was also the abundant vegetables, fruits, grains, and fish that supported the Mediterranean region—all the foods we now know to be protective of the heart. But the oil figured in. As the star flavor-maker of a healthy Mediterranean diet, olive oil is 72 percent unsaturated, so it's working at unclogging arteries even while it's imparting its magic to great dishes. Olive oil is also a good source of antioxidant vitamin E, which is not that easy to come by in the ordinary fat-conscious diet. The antioxidant "package" of vitamins, including vitamin E, cleans up those free radicals responsible for many of the destructive aspects of aging.

Compared to other fats, olive oil is uniquely protective of the stomach. It has inhibited ulcers in animal experiments and increased the gastric alkaline secretion in humans. Olive oil also may play a part in averting gallstones, especially cholesterol gallstones, because it activates bile flow and raises the helpful HDL cholesterol. And olive oil is a blood thinner that defends against strokes.

A perfect oil for sautéing, a little olive oil intensifies the flavor of the accompanying vegetables and herbs. The best all-purpose olive oil is described as "100 percent pure" on the label. It's a combination of refined olive oil and virgin olive oil. Virgin olive oil, processed with gentle filtration to remove sediments, has only 2 percent acidity and a full-bodied taste and aroma. Extra-virgin has only 1 percent acidity. So trendy has extra-virgin become that culinary aficionados hold "olive oil tastings," similar to wine tastings, and some upscale restaurants serve a small bowl of olive oil instead of butter with the bread basket. Extra-virgin olive oil is pricey, but it's even richer in omega-3s than the simple "pure." It's best saved for salads where its pronounced olive flavor is most beneficial.

Walnut Oil

Like walnuts, walnut oil is rich in omega-3 fatty acids. If you're not getting your omega-3s from fish, walnut oil would make an excellent compensatory addition to your salad oils. Might as well toss in a few walnut halves, too!

A mildly nutty flavor makes this oil a great choice for salads, whereas its low smoking point rules it out for frying. Once the bottle is opened, store walnut oil in the refrigerator.

The Anti-Aging Dairy Products

Few other foods provide the calcium boost that dairy foods do—calcium you need to keep your bones strong. Although fear of dietary fat has caused many people to veer away from milk and its products, there are some super dairy foods that deserve to be part of an anti-aging diet.

Without dairy in one's diet (or supplements), it's difficult to get the recommended amount of calcium from vegetable sources alone. Calcium, of course, is vital in preventing osteoporosis and also in keeping blood pressure in check, but these are not the only health benefits in dairy foods. Recent research has turned up a link between low calcium consumption and colon cancer.

Dairy foods are also a rich source of vitamin D, another important bone nutrient. Besides lessening the risk of broken bones as we get older, vitamin D appeared in new studies to slow or regress the progress of osteoarthritis of the knee, a condition that causes pain and restricts the activities of millions of older Americans.

Milk and milk products are an easy-to-eat source of vitamin B_{12} and protein, especially for vegetarians who have not excluded dairy foods. It would seem in this country of burgers and steaks that most people are already consuming sufficient protein, but new research has found that many Americans over the age of fifty-five are losing muscle strength and compromising their immune systems simply because they are not fulfilling their RDA for protein.

Low-fat milk and cheeses are widely available so that you can profit from the health benefits of dairy foods while keeping down that fat count.

Milk—It's Not Just for Kids Anymore

Low-fat and skim milk have caught on with the fat-conscious food buyer so well that many now find whole milk "too rich" for their taste—it's just a matter of getting used to the flavor of the new slimmed-down milk. You won't lose anything nutritionally from this switch. When the fat is skimmed off, milk is actually higher in calcium. And calcium is a vital component of an active lifestyle in later years, protecting against bone breaks and fractures and helping to keep blood pressure under control.

Some adults find they are lactose intolerant, meaning they lack lactase, an intestinal enzyme that helps to digest milk sugar (lactose). If these people consume milk or fresh cheese, the result is intestinal distress in the form of gas, bloating, and even diarrhea. But there are countermeasures that bring relief to the lactose intolerant. Lactose-reduced milk is available, or the missing enzyme can be supplied in pill form (one brand name is Lactaid®). It's also important to take dairy products with meals and not on an empty stomach.

In cooking, you'll find there are a few sauces and puddings that need whole milk if they are not to taste flat, especially when they are being made without the usual butter. But many other sauces can be enriched instead with nonfat dry milk for a "creamier" taste and for a big boost in calcium—290 milligrams in ¼ cup. You'll find many recipes in this book that call for this super ingredient.

Whole milk contains 150 calories for 8 ounces; skim milk, only 86 calories. Nonfat dry milk adds 109 calories per ¼ cup (the equivalent of 8 ounces of liquid milk).

Cheese—Varied and Versatile

High in protein and calcium, but unfortunately also high in fat and sodium, the traditional cheeses can be used sparingly as flavoring agents in a variety of vegetable dishes. Cheese is such a popular food, we can feel assured that commercial-product developers are working hard to develop low-fat substitutes for cheese lovers to buy. So far, those experts seem to be most successful with the fresh cheeses, such as ricotta, cottage, farmer's cheese, and even mozzarella. Aged cheeses with reduced fat, however, tend to be rubbery in texture and flat in flavor. Personally, I routinely choose low-fat fresh cheeses, but when it comes to a hard cheese, such as Cheddar, I'd rather cook with an ounce of the real thing than a big slab of the ersatz stuff.

Hard cheese has been shown to fight tooth decay, but as yet, no one knows how or why. Studies have shown that something in cheese counteracts the decay-causing action of sugar in the mouth.

Most nutritious of all the low-fat cheeses is the yogurt "cheese" you can make with nonfat yogurt. It has a sharper taste than cream cheese, however, and needs to be flavored with herbs and spices (see page 334).

Yogurt—a Lively Health Food

At least, it should be lively. You want to be sure to buy yogurt labeled with "active cultures" in order to take advantage of some of its unique health benefits. Although researchers may differ about the many health claims made for yogurt, there is general agreement that yogurt is helpful in preventing vaginal yeast infections. Other possible benefits include helping to relieve diarrhea (especially diarrhea caused by treatment with antibiotics) and strengthening the immune system.

In any case, yogurt definitely offers great calcium, high-quality protein, and a very convenient snack or small lunch on a busy day. And yogurt is very low in lactose, allowing many lactose-intolerant people to take advantage of milk's valuable nutrients.

Whole plain yogurt contains 139 calories for 8 ounces, with 7.4 grams of fat; nonfat yogurt is a little less, 120 calories, with no fat grams.

The Anti-Aging Animal Foods

Less meat—and leaner and lighter meat—is the right way to plan menus for a long, healthy life. At the same time, we need certain nutrients that animal foods provide more abundantly than plant foods do. The vegetarian diet, because it's plentiful in fruits and vegetables, promotes a cancer-preventing lifestyle, but it does require careful planning to supply certain other nutrients, such as protein and vitamin B_{12}, which animal foods yield abundantly.

In the case of vitamin B_{12}, animal foods, including dairy products, are the only food source, and irreversible neurological damage can result from a serious deficiency. This is not to say that you can't be a healthy vegetarian—as long as you include some dairy foods, which are also animal foods, in your diet. Total vegans, who eat no eggs, milk, meat, or fish, should obtain vitamin B_{12} from a supplement.

Surprisingly, nutritional studies have shown that some people over the age of fifty-five are not getting enough protein. Your need for protein is based on what you weigh: 0.36 grams for each pound. A person weighing 140 pounds, for instance, would need about 50 grams of protein a day. To give you an idea of how much this is in actual food, 1 cup brown rice gives you 5 grams of protein; 1 cup broccoli, 5 grams; 1 cup beans, 14 grams, 8 ounces of lowfat milk, 8 grams; 8 ounces of lowfat yogurt, 11 grams; 1 large egg, 6.3 grams; 3.5 ounces of fish, about 20 grams; 3.5 ounces of chicken, white meat without skin, 29 grams; 3.5 ounces of lean ground beef, broiled, 25 grams. As you can see from this list, you'll probably get all the protein you need from two helpings of animal foods, whereas achieving the same with plant foods will require some strategic menus.

What's the problem with those low-protein days? Those who continually undercut their protein requirement will compromise their immune system and have less energy. And high on the list of things we need as the years progress are more energy and an immune system that's in fighting trim.

The animal foods that are super nutritious are skinless poultry, especially lean turkey, and seafood, especially the so-called "oily" fish. Besides B_{12}, these supply a whole range of B vitamins, which boost brain power, strengthen the nervous system, and protect against the diseases of aging. Substituting poultry and fish for red meat is a good health move. Among other benefits, the Nurses' Health Study at the Harvard Medical School revealed that women who ate less red meat had less risk of colon cancer.

Poultry and seafood also supply us with essential fatty acids (EFAs), which are key components of the body, bringing oxygen to our tissues; keeping hair, nails, and skin younger-looking longer; and helping to prevent many degenerative diseases. There are two kinds of EFAs: omega-6s and omega-3s. Our bodies require a 2:1 ratio, twice as many omega-6s as omega-3s. In actuality, however, the usual American diet is too high in omega-6s (from animal fat) and too low in omega-3s (from fish oil).

Seafood

Seafood differs from other animal foods because it's rich in omega-3 fatty acids, whereas chicken and beef supply omega-6 fatty acids. The polyunsaturated omega-3s (eicosapentaenoic acid or EPA, and docosahexaenoic acid or DHA) have some special heart-healthy properties: They keep the blood thin, preventing the formation of clots and thus lowering the likelihood of strokes; and they reduce the amount of cholesterol the liver manufactures. The oilier the fish—which simply means that the oils are distributed throughout the flesh and not concentrated in the liver—the more omega-3s. Although you can take fish-oil supplements, overdosing may cause excessive bleeding. Nutritionists are in general agreement that the wisest course is to eat the fish that are high in omega-3s (or if those are not your favorites, at least eat some fish). How often? The most recent studies have suggested that two fish meals a week are sufficient and offer as much protection as five or six.

Early studies showed that symptoms of rheumatoid arthritis may be relieved by eating lots of fish high in omega-3 fatty acids. More recent research has suggested that the risk of developing the disease in the first place may be lower for those who eat baked or broiled fish weekly. In one study, women who ate two servings per week were 43 percent less likely to develop this painful disease.

Many kinds of fish—swordfish, lobster, salmon, shrimp, oysters, and haddock—contain a good supply of selenium, a trace mineral that works in tandem with vitamin E to lower the risk of cancer and other diseases.

Folklore has always credited fish with being good "brain food," and there's a nugget of truth there. A protein-rich meal featuring fish fills your bloodstream with tyrosine (and other amino acids). Crossing a protective filter called the blood-brain barrier, tyrosine is converted into the "alertness" chemicals dopamine and norepinephrine. That same helping of fish also supplies you with choline, which improves memory. And the omega-3s are nourishers of the brain as well as defenders of the body. No doubt about it—you'll be smart to eat fish!

Fish with the most omega-3s (but all fish contain some) are anchovies, bluefish, halibut, mackerel, pollock, salmon, sardines, swordfish, trout, and tuna.

Shellfish

In much of the earlier research into the connection between cholesterol and heart disease, shellfish suffered from bad press because they seemed to be high in cholesterol. More recently, shellfish have been returned to nutritional favor. Newer cholesterol-measuring techniques have found that certain fats in shellfish are only similar to cholesterol, and that the actual tally finds them to be lower in true cholesterol than skinless poultry. And shellfish offer many health benefits that make them a desirable part of an antiaging diet.

Shellfish are generally low in calories (compared to other animal foods) and high in protein, B vitamins, iron, zinc, copper, and iodine, as well as those protective omega-3 fatty acids. Oysters and clams are particularly rich in zinc, a mineral that not only strengthens the immune system but also plays a part in making sperm and producing male hormones.

Shellfish rich in omega-3s are clams, crab, mussels, scallops, and shrimp.

Herbs, Spices, and Teas Count for More Than Flavor

Your Spice Shelf Is a Second Medicine Chest

It's amazing to realize the many medicinal qualities of the herbs and spices we use every day to flavor our foods. Potent in prevention as well as pungent in taste, they add their influence to our defensive package of nutrients. Here are some herbal highlights.

Essential oils obtained from thyme and oregano inhibit the invasions of bacteria and fungus. Saffron shows an antioxidant and antitumor activity. It's one of the costliest spices, but it only takes a few brilliant threads of saffron to flavor a whole dish. Turmeric (sometimes called "poor man's saffron," because it colors a dish the same lush golden-yellow) has anti-inflammatory properties, and both turmeric and cumin inhibit blood clotting. Cumin, poppy seeds, turmeric, and basil have been shown likely to suppress carcinogenesis, or, in other words, to stop cancers before they get started. Rosemary contains many powerful antioxidants, which have been found to prevent cancer in animal studies, and also a pinch of heart-healthy minerals such as calcium, magnesium, and potassium. Cayenne pepper is linked to the health of cardiovascular and respiratory systems. Paprika and chili powder are moderate sources of beta-carotene. Allspice and cloves are local anesthetics, first aid for pain of tooth and gum. Anise, fennel, caraway, coriander, and dill are all considered to be digestive aids. Celery seed is a diuretic and a deterrent to high blood pressure. Another diuretic, parsley, is high in antioxidants that neutralize carcinogens and is a breath freshener whose essential oil is an ingredient in over-the-counter preparations for keeping the breath sweet. Fenugreek, often included in curry powders, is antidiarrheal and antiulcer, and helps to control intestinal gas. It's also antidiabetic, helping to lower blood sugar, and is a cholesterol-lowering agent as well. Besides its long and honorable folkloric history as a medicine dating back to the ancient Egyptians, fenugreek was the chief ingredient, other than alcohol, in a popular remedy for "female complaints" of the past century.

Sage Advice on Carminative Herbs

If you'd like to include more legumes in your daily diet but fear their intestinal effects, season them with the herbs and spices that are carminatives, that is, those that relax the stomach, absorb intestinal gas, and reduce flatulence. By a happy coincidence, they're some of the very flavors that harmonize well with beans: caraway, cardamom, coriander, dill, ginger, sage, and thyme.

Potent Ginger—a Multimedicinal

Strong in flavor and in medicinal action, ginger is an antinausea agent that has been shown to work as well as a leading over-the-counter drug for motion sickness. If you enjoy the peppery "grown-up" flavor of crystallized ginger, it might be just the right "candy" to take with you on trips. Arthritis sufferers should find some relief from pain and swelling in ginger, which inhibits prostaglandins the same way as many of the anti-inflammatory drugs. Ginger, along with garlic, is reported to make platelets less likely to stick and clog arteries. It's also rich in melatonin, a wonder nutrient that helps you to sleep while it revs up your defense against free radicals.

You wouldn't want to eat gingerbread every day, but a pleasant way to enjoy ginger on a daily basis is to fix yourself a nice relaxing cup of ginger tea (page 313) or mix up some Ginger Sugar (page 338) to sprinkle on cereal, toast, or muffins.

A Nice Cup of Tea Is Good for What Ails You

The world's most popular beverage has gained the attention of nutrition researchers in both hemispheres. Early Asian studies seemed to show a connection between green tea and protection from cancer. Later studies in the West, however, came up with comparable results when black tea was included. Teas of the nonherbal variety—whether green, black, or oolong (which is somewhere between green and black)—contain potent anticancer chemicals called polyphenols. Many studies have revealed that research animals given tea with their drinking water have a reduced risk of developing tumors of the esophagus, colon, liver, pancreas, and breast. Benign lumps were less likely to become cancerous. Protection against skin cancer has also been shown for tea-drinking mice who were given the equivalent of four cups a day.

One caution: Drinking very hot tea (130 to 150F; 55 to 65C) over a period of time damages the windpipe and *increases* the risk of esophageal cancer.

Tea's hearty brew also reduces LDL cholesterol and inhibits blood clotting. In a major twenty-five-year study of tea drinkers in seven different countries, there was a moderately reduced risk of death from coronary heart disease.

THE ANTI-AGING ARSENAL

We live in an age when good nutrition is finally being recognized by the scientific community as a viable way of preventing disease, maintaining youthfulness, and prolonging life. Many studies of the eating habits of people in all areas of the world have revealed a promising relationship between healthy food choices and less risk of disease. Follow-up animal studies have confirmed that food can be a first defense against heart disease and cancer. The good news that our heart health is improving has been credited, in part, to better eating habits and overall nutrition savvy. The National Cancer Institute now asserts that one-third of all cancer deaths may be related to what foods are consumed, and we are urged to include plenty of known anticancer foods in our daily diets. In a recent summary that appeared in the *Journal of the American Dietetic Association,* a review of the scientific literature from 206 human epidemiologic studies and 22 animal studies confirmed the protective effect of eating more fruits and vegetables against a variety of cancers. The highest protective association was attributed to allium vegetables (garlic, onion, etc.), carrots, green vegetables, cruciferous vegetables (broccoli, cabbage, etc.) and tomatoes, with 70 percent or more of the studies yielding positive results for these foods.

Choosing the nutritional superfoods is something easy and enjoyable you can do for your health and youthfulness every day.

What follows is a summary of our current arsenal against the disorders and diseases of aging.

Antioxidants—Our Old Friends Vitamins A, C, and E

In recent years you've heard a great deal about antioxidants—chemicals that keep other substances from being oxidized. Rust on an old metal is a good example of unchecked oxidation. Fruit slices turning brown or fats rancid are others. Because you breathe oxygen, your body is in the same danger of oxidation as the body of an aging car.

But when you consume sufficient antioxidants (probably at higher than the suggested minimum daily requirements), they work to clean up the accumulation of runaway free radicals, unstable and highly reactive, ready to bond with other molecules and cause random damage. Spewed out from every biological process, free radicals in excess can lead to cellular and DNA damage—and to cancer.

Antioxidants also prevent the oxidation of LDL cholesterol, which scientists now believe to be the culprit that clogs arteries. Two of the antioxidant vitamins, C and E, have a beneficial effect on the carotid artery walls, reversing the thickness that occurs with fatty deposits and reducing the risk of stroke. In defending you against free radicals, antioxidants are protecting you against the ravages of age—a kind of vitamin "fountain of youth."

There's nothing exotic about antioxidant superfoods; they're common everyday fruits, vegetables, grains, and oils. The National Cancer Institute especially recommends the whole foods containing antioxidant nutrients, rather than supplements, to reduce the risk of various cancers. In recent, disappointing studies, some antioxidant supplements, such as beta-carotene (precursor to vitamin A), have not been as effective as the foods themselves. Although it's easy enough with a little planning to consume plenty of vitamins A and C—a sweet potato and a kiwifruit would put you way over the top of your RDA (which is where you should be)—it's much harder to obtain enough vitamin E without the use of supplements, because the best sources are calorie-rich oils, nuts, seeds, and wheat germ.

Vital Vitamin A

Nature gives us vitamin A in two ways. Preformed vitamin A is found in all animal foods, of which the richest source is fish oil. Your body can use preformed vitamin A "as is," but it has to convert the low-fat vegetable version, called provitamin or precursor vitamin A. Since vegetables and fruits contain no saturated fats, there's an advantage to getting your vitamin A from plant foods.

The marvelous carotenoids are vegetable precursors of vitamin A, and what a protective package they are! Anti-aging vitamin A is vital to maintaining cell membranes. It helps to care for your skin, hair, nails, teeth, gums, and bones, and it's essential to the overall health of your eyes, in addition to preventing night blindness.

Vitamin A is critical to the immune function, and it protects against cancers of the esophagus, larynx, lung, and prostate.

VITAMIN A SUPERFOODS

Orange fruits: apricots, cantaloupe, mangoes, nectarines, papayas, and peaches
Greens, the darker the better
Red bell peppers and red chiles
Orange vegetables: carrots, sweet potatoes, butternut squash, pumpkin
Seafood

Vitamin C—the Great Healer

An essential nutrient for the immune system, vitamin C helps your body resist infections of all kinds. It's important to the healing of cuts and wounds, so you ought to have plenty of vitamin C in your system when you undergo any kind of medical procedure. It protects against cancers of the esophagus, stomach, and pancreas.

Vitamin C is necessary to heart health as well. It lowers the harmful LDL cholesterol and raises the helpful HDL cholesterol. It strengthens artery walls, and helps to keep them free of fatty deposits.

Arthritis progresses more slowly in people who consume 150 to 180 milligrams of vitamin C daily, perhaps because it's important to collagen, and collagen is a large part of cartilage. Collagen is also vital to a youthful skin, as you will note if

you read the claims of various skin creams.

VITAMIN C SUPERFOODS

Berries: strawberries, raspberries, fresh black currants
Broccoli
Cabbage and brussels sprouts
Citrus fruits: grapefruit, oranges, tangerines
Kale
Kiwifruit
Melons
Parsley
Potatoes
Tomatoes

Vitamin E—Protection for Body and Brain

Especially notable for its contribution to heart health, vitamin E has been shown in many major tests to reduce substantially the occurrence of heart disease in men and women who have taken from 100 to 250 International Units (IU) daily for two years. This is one incidence in which supplements proved to be as effective as whole foods. But whether or not you take a supplement, including vitamin E–rich foods in your meals is nutritional insurance against heart disease and many other undesirable encroachments of age.

Vitamin E (in substantial amounts) has shown promise in relieving the pain and swelling of arthritis. This antioxidant is also a big booster of the immune system. High blood levels of vitamin E seem to protect against cancers of the colon, mouth, throat, and lung.

Those brown spots on hand and face that are associated with aging are caused by the pigment lipofuscin, which is also believed to be connected, less visibly, to senility. The accumulation of lipofuscin in the tissues is lessened by a high intake of vitamin E. Some scientists believe that vitamin E improves circulation to the brain and lessens the occurrence of age-related mental disorders while it's staving off those dark patches on your skin. All this adds up to a lot of great reasons for keeping up on vitamin E nutrition.

VITAMIN E SUPERFOODS

Asparagus

Avocados

Brussels sprouts

Leafy greens: kale, spinach

Nuts and seeds

Oils: soybean, sesame, sunflower, peanut, flaxseed, olive

Mangoes

Tomatoes

Seafood: halibut, lobster

Whole grains: whole wheat, wheat germ, whole oats, whole-wheat couscous

B Is for Brain Power—and Much More!

In our stressful times, what could be more important than the B vitamins? Taken as a package (B complex), they are vital to the normal functioning of the brain and nervous system. A wide range of studies has shown that B vitamins keep the mind healthy, enhance the immune system, help to ward off cancer and coronary disease, and prevent some birth defects. Because they are water soluble, the B vitamins must constantly be replaced. And the need for some B vitamins—B_6 and B_{12}—increases as we get older. Unfortunately, the typical American diet is lacking in at least two key Bs, folate and B_6. Many women consume only half their RDA of B_6.

A high concentration of the amino acid homocysteine in the blood is considered a warning of future heart disease. It's been discovered, however, that three of the B vitamins—folate, B_6, and B_{12}—decrease the concentration of homocysteine and therefore lessen the risk of clogged arteries, stroke, and heart attacks. The body needs all three to convert homocysteine to less dangerous substances, but folate is the key player.

B_6 and B_{12} also help to prevent the impairment of the nervous system that comes with advancing years. A deficiency in folate, B_6, and B_{12} adversely influences cognitive abilities such as perception, memory, judgment, reasoning, and even spatial skills like drawing in perspective. A thiamine (B_1) deficiency can cause severe chronic memory problems. To combat stress, sleeplessness and even jet lag, niacin (B_3) and B_6 promote the conversion of tryptophan to serotonin to melatonin.

Don't be tempted to take only one or two of the B vitamins in supplement form, because an overdose in one B vitamin can cause a deficiency in another. This is not a mistake that nature makes; the big B vitamin foods, like beans and whole grains, provide several in one package.

Perk Up with Thiamine (B₁) Superfoods

If you want to feel energetic, eat plenty of these foods. Thiamine is connected to the metabolism of carbohydrates, making it a vitalizer vitamin. It also contributes to the overall B-complex package that strengthens the entire nervous system.

Maturity may bring wisdom, but it also brings those annoying little lapses in memory we would all prefer to avoid. But thiamine protects memory, so *never forget* to put the following foods on your shopping list!

Broccoli
Brussels sprouts
Citrus fruits
Corn
Dates and figs
Legumes: beans and peas
Mangoes
Nuts and seeds
Pineapple
Seafood
Watermelon
Wheat germ and whole-grain foods
Winter squash

Stay Vigorous with Riboflavin (B₂) Superfoods

If you exercise regularly (even walk or garden or house-clean vigorously), you need to include riboflavin, the fitness vitamin, in your daily fare. It's particularly effective at sponging up those extra free radicals spewed out by strenuous workouts, whether jogging or cleaning out the garage.

A deficiency in riboflavin can cause chapped lips, sores on the tongue, and vision problems in older adults.

Beet greens
Broccoli
Low-fat dairy products
Mushrooms
Nuts: almonds, cashews, walnuts
Sweet potatoes
Poultry
Pumpkin
Seafood and shellfish
Spinach
Wheat germ and whole-grain foods

Treat Your Heart Right with Niacin (B₃) Superfoods

Niacin is the B vitamin that's often prescribed (at high doses) to lower cholesterol, so you know that including niacin superfoods in your menus is a step in the right direction. In addition, niacin is needed for building strong nerves, the body's message service, and for the proper formation of DNA.

Apricots
Bananas
Barley
Brown rice
Mangoes

Mushrooms

Nuts: almonds, chestnuts, peanuts

Potatoes

Seafood and shellfish

Sunflower seeds

Poultry

Wheat germ and whole-grain foods

Feel Good with Pyridoxine (B₆)
Superfoods

Fight off those passing viruses and bacteria! Animal studies have shown that pyridoxine boosts immunity. It also defends the body by slowing the growth of tumors, including skin cancers.

Even a slight deficiency in pyridoxine sends your nervous system into a panic and may be responsible for confusion and depression. Unfortunately, most people aren't getting enough pyridoxine from their ordinary meals. So, if you ever feel blue for no good reason, start stocking up on the following.

Avocados

Bananas

Carrots

Dried fruits: apricots, currants, prunes, raisins

Legumes: lentils

Nuts: chestnuts, filberts, peanuts, walnuts

Poultry

Seafood and shellfish

Soybeans

Sunflower seeds

Sweet potatoes

Watermelon

Wheat germ and whole-grain foods

Winter squash

Fabulous Folate (Folic Acid, Folacin)
Superfoods

Scientists have been trying to pinpoint what it is about a diet rich in fruits and vegetables and low in fats that offers such significant protection against colon cancer. One possibility is the combination of folate with other vitamins, phytochemicals, and fiber, because people who eat the folate foods are less likely to develop this form of cancer. In animal studies, too, even mild deprivation of folate resulted in colorectal tumors. This may be because folate has a direct effect on DNA, and errors in DNA are thought to trigger cancer. Folate also protects against birth defects.

Folate protects against stroke and heart attack by decreasing high homocysteine in the blood.

The only problem with folate is that having a good supply can mask the nerve-degenerative symptoms of a deficiency in vitamin B_{12}. This deficiency is a special danger to vegans, who eat no animal foods at all, and to the elderly, who may not metabolize B_{12} well enough. That means, if you're getting enough folate, you need to be sure you're also getting plenty of vitamin B_{12}. The B vitamins always perform best in concert.

SUPERFOOD SOURCES OF FOLATE

Asparagus

Avocados

Barley
Beets
Broccoli
Brussels sprouts
Cabbage
Cauliflower
Corn
Greens, dark leafy
Legumes: beans and peas
Nuts and seeds
Oranges
Plantains
Whole grains

Vitamin B_{12} Superfoods to Stay Mentally Alert

This important vitamin is made from bacteria found only in animal foods or in a few fermented soy products, such as soy sauce. Vegetarians who include dairy products and/or eggs in their diets will be getting B_{12} in the bargain. Vegans who eat only plant foods ought to consume some vital B_{12} or take a supplement. Why is it such a worry? A deficiency of B_{12} can cause the whole range of mental problems associated with aging and ascribed (sometimes incorrectly) to senility. Severe memory loss, mental confusion, delusions, nerve damage, and even psychosis have sometimes been traced to a low level of B_{12}.

VITAMIN B_{12} SUPERFOODS

Low-fat dairy products
Poultry
Seafood and shellfish

Vitamin D Keeps You Kicking

Older adults are often vitamin-D deficient, especially those who don't get outdoors. Although vitamin D is a nutrient that can be obtained from food, it's also manufactured by exposure to daylight. Just take a walk "on the sunny side of the street" for ten to fifteen minutes three times a week to fulfill your RDA. But you may want to do better than that. Recent research into older adults with arthritic knees found that a low level of vitamin D in the blood correlated with a reduced ability to repair the damage that arthritis does to bones and cartilage. So maintain an adequate intake of vitamin D to keep your knees in good shape.

VITAMIN D SUPERFOODS

Milk and milk products fortified with
    vitamin D
Seafood: salmon, sardines, shrimp, oysters

Carbohydrates—the Comforting Staff of Life

Carbohydrates come in two forms, simple and complex. Simple carbohydrates are the "sweets," from plain table sugar to honey and molasses. Complex carbohydrates are the starches found in grains and vegetables such as beans and potatoes, which also contain the important vitamins, minerals, and fiber that sweets lack. Happily, vegetables and fruits rich in complex carbohydrates also have a high water content and relatively few calories. While their bulk helps to satisfy your appetite, they're also good foods for keeping weight under control. Complex carbohydrates form the broad base of the food pyramid, and six to eleven servings a day are recommended. These are the foods that sustain physical and mental energy for work and play, as they have sustained the energy of generations before us. Athletes still stock up on carbs for peak performance in competition.

The National Cancer Institute recommends that we increase the amount of starches as well as fiber in our diets by eating more complex-carbohydrate foods. Literally hundreds of studies have found that diets high in these foods reduce the risk of cancer. Many complex-carbohydrate foods are rich in soluble fiber, a heart saver that reduces blood cholesterol. These are foods we need to combat the diseases of aging.

Keep calm with the good carbs! Carbohydrate foods have been shown to affect our emotional behavior. They raise the level of serotonin, a neurotransmitter that plays an important role in mood states and appetite control. Low levels of serotonin are associated with anxiety, depression, and migraine headaches. High levels promote a reduction in tension and produce a sense of well-being. Since some of the leading antidepressant drugs work by raising or maintaining the level of serotonin in the brain, carbohydrates legitimately may be called a natural antidepressant—and are inexpensive and tasty to

boot! The effect is more pronounced if the carbohydrate food is eaten without any accompanying protein. Serotonin is also a precursor of melatonin, which helps to achieve a more tranquil state of mind, plus all its other benefits of slowed aging and increased vitality.

There is also some indication that serotonin has an effect on reducing fat intake, normalizing appetite, and discouraging binge eating. Prozac, the antidepressant drug that increases serotonin in the brain, has had the side effect of weight loss.

A note about carbo-phobia. A spate of recent diet books has made carbohydrates the culprit in weight gain. Some of these carbo-bashing diets work, simply because you consume fewer calories when you drastically cut down on the big carbohydrate foods: fruits, vegetables, breads, and pasta. For one thing, high-protein and low-carb diets cause a loss in appetite (and also cause bad breath, constipation, and even gout if uric acid levels soar too high). You lose weight, but you also lose the vitamins, minerals, phytochemicals, and fiber that are essential to staying energetic, mentally fit, and healthy. Alas, the best way to lose weight is still simply to eat a well-rounded diet but less of it, with an emphasis on low-fat foods. One gram of carbohydrates has only 4 calories as compared to 9 calories in a gram of fat. Naturally, you have to get more exercise, too. To lose weight, the bottom line has to read: *more energy expended than consumed*. But moderation never generates the high excitement of a drastic diet plan, whatever that plan may be at the moment.

COMPLEX-CARBOHYDRATE SUPERFOODS

Bananas
Barley
Corn and cornmeal
Legumes: beans and peas
Mangoes
Oats
Papayas
Pasta
Potatoes
Rice
Squash
Whole-grain baked goods and cereals

Always Remember Choline!

A memory nutrient that's very much like a B vitamin, choline is a component of lecithin, a fatlike substance that occurs in some foods. Choline is used by the body to manufacture acetylcholine, a neurotransmitter that's critical to memory, to the formation of the membranes around nerve fibers, and to many other biological processes. Scientists give the choline-memory connection mixed reviews, but there is a body of evidence that choline-rich foods may give memory power a boost.

While your body manufactures choline with the assistance of B vitamins, higher levels may improve memory or at least help to avoid age-related memory loss. One of the best sources of choline is egg yolk. Although eggs are high in cholesterol and not included in the superfoods list, the American Heart Association affirms that people whose cholesterol levels are normal may include three to four eggs in their weekly diets. If you do enjoy eggs, you'll be benefiting from the choline they contain.

SUPERFOOD SOURCES OF CHOLINE

Nuts: pecans, peanuts
Oatmeal
Rice
Seafood
Soybeans
Wheat germ and wheat products

Melatonin—More Calm and Comfort from Food

The principal hormone produced by the pineal gland, an organ in the brain's center, melatonin has many useful functions in the body, and more are being discovered every day. Here's what we know now: Melatonin enhances restful sleep, boosts the immune system, defends against aging by mopping up free radicals that can damage cells, relieves stress, increases vitality, and reduces the effects of jet lag by helping to keep the body's circadian rhythm synchronized with the twenty-four-hour cycle. The body manufactures melatonin every night during sleep, but as we add on the years, melatonin production can slow down, just when we need it most. Scientists speculate that this waning in melatonin may be the reason for the higher incidence of insomnia among seniors. Many people who've read about the wonders of melatonin have rushed out to buy supplements, but actually there are good sources of melatonin among the superfoods.

SUPERFOOD SOURCES OF MELATONIN

Bananas
Corn
Ginger
Oats
Rice
Tomatoes

Mineral Magic

Boron—a Bone and Brain Mineral

This trace mineral found in plant foods doesn't get much media attention, although it's essential to the efficient absorption of calcium for strong bones. That makes boron an osteoporosis fighter, and it may be instrumental in helping to relieve arthritis as well.

Boron is also a brain booster, increasing alertness and the ability to learn. Researchers have found that low boron levels can impair memory and motor skills. All in all, to stay bright and active through the years, keep boron foods on the menu.

SUPERFOOD SOURCES OF BORON

Apples
Broccoli
Carrots
Dark, leafy greens
Dried fruits: prunes, raisins, dates
Grapes
Honey

Legumes: beans and peas
Nuts: almonds, hazelnuts, peanuts
Peaches
Pears

Calcium to Keep Straight and Strong

As you add years, your calcium needs increase, and yet often the very dairy products that are the chief source of dietary calcium are gradually given up for one reason or another—fear of fat or lactose intolerance, for instance. Yet calcium is essential to preventing osteoporosis, the gradual bone thinning that is the most common skeletal disorder in the United States and a major health problem for many older women and some men, affecting an estimated 24 million people. Not only do bones become more fragile, but people also grow shorter because of collapsed vertebrae. Well-designed studies have clearly shown that bone loss can be slowed by sufficient calcium. Yet USDA surveys show that most people are not getting the recommended amount. Women, who are most at risk for osteoporosis, average even less than men. Dairy foods are still the best source of calcium because they also provide the vitamin D, protein, and zinc needed for normal bone metabolism.

Not all the calcium in foods is absorbed: A glass of skim milk, for example, contains 300 milligrams of calcium, but you probably absorb only 20 to 40 percent of it. Absorption is always improved, however, if you eat a food containing vitamin C in the same meal. This can be easy and pleasant. Think of low-fat mozzarella accompanied by sliced ripe tomatoes and basil!

Even when eating good whole foods, you may find you also need to take supplements to fulfill your daily requirement. Calcium citrate is recommended by many nutritionists as being easily assimilated and digested. Calcium carbonate (the chief ingredient in a leading antacid tablet) also reduces stomach acid. But some older people don't produce enough stomach acid to digest protein foods properly, which causes a different kind of indigestion, so constantly suppressing stomach acid is not desirable for them.

Recent research has suggested that besides its value in keeping you straight and strong, calcium also helps to regulate blood pressure at all ages, even in children. It seems to work best, however, on those whose high blood pressure is sodium sensitive. And there is evidence that calcium protects against colon cancer.

SUPERFOOD SOURCES OF CALCIUM

Broccoli

Dairy products: low-fat milk, nonfat yogurt, cheese

Canned fish with bones: salmon, sardines

Dark, leafy greens

Molasses

Soybeans and tofu

Chromium—an Important Regulator

Hypoglycemia (too little blood sugar) or diabetes (too high blood sugar)—no matter which way the metabolism swings, nutritionists report that improved chromium nutrition leads to improved sugar metabolism. This is not to say that chromium is a cure for diabetes, but it's the mineral that helps to maintain normal glucose tolerance. This is an important factor as we get older and problems with insulin are liable to occur.

Almost 95 percent of diabetics have Type II Diabetes Mellitus (non-insulin-dependent diabetes), an adult-onset disorder in which people have trouble removing sugar from their blood. When blood sugar or glucose is produced from the food we eat, the pancreas secretes insulin, which enables glucose to pass into the cells, where it's stored, or burned to produce energy. If for some reason a person's insulin loses its effectiveness or not enough insulin is produced, the body has trouble clearing glucose out of the bloodstream. This results in high levels of glucose in the blood that spills over into the urine. There are many complications of diabetes, some of them life-threatening. Diabetes is the fourth leading cause of death in the United States.

Since chromium also regulates cholesterol and fatty acid production in the liver, a deficiency may contribute to atherosclerosis.

Unfortunately, chromium is poorly absorbed, so it's important to include a variety of chromium superfoods in your weekly menus. The chromium in animal foods and whole-grain foods is the most easily assimilated, but all of the following superfoods will enhance your body's store of this vital mineral.

SUPERFOOD SOURCES OF CHROMIUM

Apples, unpeeled
Barley
Broccoli
Grapes, grape juice, raisins
Green beans
Mushrooms
Nuts
Potatoes with skins
Shellfish
Turkey
Wheat germ, cereals, and bread

Copper—a Blood Builder

A diet rich in whole grains and legumes should fulfill the body's needs for copper. It's needed to heal wounds and to manufacture red blood cells, bones, and collagen, which is so important to keeping skin supple. Copper is also vital to respiration because it helps in the synthesis of hemoglobin, the part of the blood that carries oxygen. Low levels of copper are linked to high blood pressure; a deficiency decreases a relaxing factor necessary to normal levels. Copper is also a blood antioxidant that works with vitamin C to protect cellular health.

Remember when folks wore copper bracelets to relieve arthritis? Perhaps it would have been more effective to consume copper-rich foods. Interestingly, copper appears to decrease the need for pain medication in arthritis and other chronic conditions.

SUPERFOOD SOURCES OF COPPER

Avocados
Legumes: beans, peas, and especially
    soybeans
Molasses
Mushrooms
Nuts: almonds, peanuts, pecans, wal-
    nuts
Shellfish: lobster, oysters
Whole-grain cereal
Whole wheat

Iron—Can You Have Too Much of a Good Thing?

Iron is vital to hemoglobin, the substance in blood that carries oxygen from the lungs to all parts of the body, so iron is involved in respiration, energy, and, in fact, life itself. Although a widely publicized 1992 study reported that high levels of iron may increase the risk of heart disease, subsequent research has not confirmed that finding. In fact, a more recent five-year study sponsored by the National Institute on Aging found that older people with the highest iron levels were less likely to die of heart disease—or from any cause.

If you're an adult male who's not a vegetarian, chances are you're already getting enough iron. It's just the opposite with women of childbearing age, who lose blood every month, and with children, who frequently do not eat enough iron-rich protein foods. These two groups often have iron-poor blood (if not actual anemia), which can lead to fatigue, listlessness, depression, and susceptibility to infection. Iron-deficient children may exhibit symptoms of attention-deficit hyperactivity.

The greatest source of easily absorbed iron is red meat, especially organ meats. If eaten at the same time, foods that contain vitamin C enhance absorption. Cooking (especially acid foods) in cast-iron pans is also a source of dietary iron. Two substances known to decrease the amount of iron absorbed from foods are high fiber and tea.

SUPERFOOD SOURCES OF IRON

Fruits, dried
Legumes: beans and peas
Molasses
Nuts
Potatoes with their skins
Poultry: turkey, chicken
Pumpkin
Sardines
Shellfish
Tofu
Tuna
Vegetables, dark green: broccoli, brussels sprouts, and leafy varieties

Magnesium—an Enzyme Activator

Maybe it doesn't get the press coverage that some of the "bigger" nutrients do, but magnesium is truly vital to an anti-aging diet. This energetic trace mineral activates the enzymes needed in literally hundreds of cellular functions, including the metabolism of carbohydrates, proteins, and fats.

In study after study, magnesium has been shown to protect against diseases and disorders that are associated with aging. Number one is its importance to a healthy heart. A deficiency in magnesium is definitely considered to be a risk factor not only for high blood pressure but also for irregular heartbeat and ischemic heart disease (obstruction of the inflow of arterial blood). Some studies have suggested that magnesium may defend against the development of asthma and other lung disorders. It works with calcium to maintain strong bones and prevent the fractures so common in later life. Magnesium is also credited with reducing tooth decay by binding calcium to tooth enamel. It's a memory agent, too; magnesium therapy has been used on patients with Alzheimer's disease.

A balanced diet that includes plenty of vegetables, fruits, and whole grains should supply sufficient magnesium. Nevertheless, the standard American diet has indeed proved to be deficient. Too many sweets or high-fat foods, or too much alcohol will compromise magnesium levels in the body. Even without these excesses, only a third of older Americans are getting all the magnesium they need.

SUPERFOOD SOURCES OF MAGNESIUM

Artichokes
Avocados
Bananas
Fish

Millet

Molasses

Nuts: almonds, Brazil nuts, hazelnuts, peanuts

Pumpkin seeds

Vegetables, dark green

Whole wheat

(A note of cheer for chocoholics: Although it's not a superfood, chocolate is a rich source of magnesium, too.)

Manganese—a Jack-of-All-Trades

An antioxidant mineral, manganese is a vital part of the defense against the degenerative course called aging and an integral part of many body processes. Among its several activities, it stimulates enzymes that help to utilize brain boosters like choline, biotin, and thiamine. It aids in the synthesis of fatty acids and cholesterol. Like boron, manganese helps in bone metabolism, so it works against osteoporosis. Since too much manganese can be toxic to the nervous system, it's best to avoid big supplement doses in favor of the good whole foods that follow.

SUPERFOOD SOURCES OF MANGANESE

Avocados

Beans

Berries: blueberries, raspberries

Nuts

Oatmeal

Pineapple and pineapple juice

Spinach

Tea

Whole-wheat and whole-grain products

Potassium—a Great Heart Protector

Potassium and sodium are teamed together in maintaining the body's fluid balance and helping to keep the heartbeat normal. High blood pressure and its damaging effect can be reduced, along with the risk of strokes, with a sufficient intake of potassium. A diet high in potassium, therefore, is a great protector of the heart. Unfortunately, the diuretics (water pills) often prescribed for high blood pressure or dieting are liable to wash the potassium out of one's system as well. A bout of diarrhea also can deplete potassium levels. Yet just one banana a day can supply nearly a quarter of one's RDA for potassium.

Potassium also plays a role in preserving normal kidney function, stimulating them to eliminate poisonous body wastes. It's vital to muscle contraction (including the heart) and nerve impulses, and it's a catalyst in carbohydrate and protein metabolism.

SUPERFOOD SOURCES OF POTASSIUM

Apples

Apricots

Asparagus

Avocados

Bananas

Broccoli

Brussels sprouts

Legumes: beans, peas

Melons

Molasses

Mushrooms

Oranges

Peaches
Potatoes
Tomatoes
Wheat germ
Yogurt

Selenium—a Super Team Player

An antioxidant team player, selenium is an essential mineral that works with vitamin E to clean up the damaging excess of free radicals that can cause the diseases and disorders of aging, from eye problems to cancer. In some promising recent research involving human subjects, selenium reduced the risk of cancers of the lung, prostate, and colon.

Selenium is necessary for the formation of prostaglandins, powerful hormonelike substances that stimulate a number of bodily functions, including blood pressure. It helps to preserve elasticity of tissue as we grow older. Some scientists think that selenium may also enhance the immune system. Too much selenium can be toxic, however, so it's best to stay with the whole foods that supply this trace mineral rather than to take supplements.

SUPERFOOD SOURCES OF SELENIUM
Asparagus
Brazil nuts
Mushrooms
Seafood and shellfish
Seeds: sesame, sunflower
Wheat germ and whole grains

Zinc to Repair and Heal

Second in abundance only to iron in the body, zinc is a trace mineral of vital importance to the activity of enzymes in countless metabolic processes. It's an antioxidant mineral, scourge of free radicals, and in general gears up the immune system against all invaders. Zinc is essential in the synthesis of DNA, which conveys inherited traits and directs each cell's activity. It's needed to speed up body repairs such as wound healing. It's a necessary component of bone building. It's important to discriminatory sharpness of taste and smell (indispensable to good cooking—and eating!). A deficiency in zinc has been implicated in male reproductive and prostate disorders. And zinc has even been cited recently as lessening the symptoms of a cold, although the jury is still out on that one.

Eating a diet rich in zinc is the way to go. Taking megadoses of zinc via supplements (unless prescribed by a physician for an actual deficiency) is not a good idea, since a zinc overload has been linked to Alzheimer's disease. Deficiencies are more liable to be found among athletes, who sweat out more zinc, and drinkers, because alcohol causes more zinc to be excreted. Strict vegetarians (vegans) may also be deficient simply because they don't eat animal foods.

Oysters are the single greatest source of zinc, with a plate of oysters on the half shell yielding as much as ten times the required amount. But no other superfood goes that far overboard.

Brown rice

Dairy products

Legumes: dried beans, peas, and lentils

Nuts: peanuts, pecans, Brazil nuts, cashews

Seeds: pumpkin, sunflower, squash

Shellfish, especially oysters

Turkey, especially dark meat

Wheat germ and whole grains

Phytochemicals: The Food Drugstore

Created not by man but by nature, these chemical compounds are the exciting new vitamins—or "phytomins"—of the future. One of the reasons whole foods seem to be more effective than supplements in preserving health and youthfulness may be because fruits and vegetables are rich in phytochemicals as well as vitamins and minerals. These newly recognized substances (also called "nutraceuticals") are biologically active nonnutrients that give a plant its characteristic color, odor, and flavor along with protection against the ravages of weather extremes and the assaults of insects. Researchers now theorize that these substances may have the ability to defend the human body as well.

The National Cancer Institute began a project in 1990 to study the effects of phytochemicals on cancers. Although scientists haven't learned exactly how they work, several phytogenic substances in foods have been found to prevent the development of certain cancers in animals.

They interfere with the progress of the disease at every stage, from blocking the formation of carcinogens to repairing damaged DNA and choking off the blood supply of cancerous cells that have formed. There are literally hundreds of thousands of phytochemicals in foods, and nutritional research has only begun to scratch the surface in discovering, classifying, and studying a comparative few. Results have been so outstanding, however, that phytochemicals have become overnight nutritional stars, not only of prevention but also of possible treatment. Here are some of the winners, and where to find them.

Allicin (or Allylic/Allyl Sulfides)—New Status for a Folk-Remedy Favorite

Credited by healers with having great medicinal and spiritual powers and revered by cooks for their culinary magic throughout the ages, the flavorsome vegetables containing allicin have been newly recognized as effective preventative medicine. Allicin foods have been found to lower LDL cholesterol and to act as blood thinners, guarding against strokes. They detoxify cancer-causing chemicals in the stomach and digestive tract. Allicin is also inimical to bacteria, viruses, and fungal infections. Be sure to cook with plenty of these delicious taste enhancers during cold and flu season!

Chives

Garlic

Leeks
Onions
Scallions

Capsaicin

Found in that delicious "hot stuff" that characterizes many ethnic dishes, capsaicin neutralizes carcinogens and also strengthens the respiratory tract against its various winter foes and woes. A nice bowl of chicken soup is known to relieve the miseries of a cold, but a few drops of hot pepper sauce will make it even more effective. Capsaicin works to cause an excess of fluids in the air passages (not to mention the tears in your eyes!). This in turn thins out mucus so that it flows more easily. Your sinuses clear; congestion breaks up; and the bronchial passages of your lungs are flushed out.

Surprisingly, these feisty, fiery foods don't cause ulcers or harm the normal stomach at all. If your mouth doesn't complain, you don't have to worry about enjoying hot chiles.

SUPERFOOD SOURCES OF CAPSAICIN
Chiles, the hotter the better

Catechins—a Cup of Prevention

Asian research into the potential benefits of green tea has revealed the power of catechins, one of the phytochemicals it contains, as an immune-system booster and, more recently, as a protector against stomach cancer. Because it inhibits the breakdown of collagen, catechin may also prove to be useful in the treatment of arthritis.

SUPERFOOD SOURCES OF CATECHINS
Berries
Tea: green and black, but not herbal

Chlorogenic Acid and P-coumaric Acid— a Potent Pair

These two phytochemicals, found in the same foods, team up to detoxify cancer-causing nitrosamines during digestion. So if you indulge in that occasional slice of ham, or in any cured meat (such as hot dogs or bacon) that causes nitrosamines to form, don't forget the complementary pineapple slice or perhaps a side order of tomato salad.

SUPERFOOD SOURCES OF CHLOROGENIC
ACID AND P-COUMARIC ACID
Peppers
Pineapple
Strawberries
Tomatoes

Indoles—an Important Defense

One of the first of the anticancer phytochemicals to be discovered, indoles stimulate enzymes that protect against common cancers such as colon, lung, esophageal, and prostate. One form of these phytochemicals, indole-3-carbinol, protects against abnormal estrogen stimulation, thereby defending against breast cancer. Indoles are found abundantly in the wonderful cruciferous vegetable family.

SUPERFOOD SOURCES OF INDOLES

Broccoli

Brussels sprouts

Cabbage

Cauliflower

Greens: collards, kale, mustard greens

Turnips and rutabaga

Sulforaphane and Other Isothiocyanates—Cancer Blockers

Found in cruciferous plants (whose leaves form a cross), sulforaphane detoxifies and removes carcinogens before they can do any harm. The compound is so stable that cooking won't diminish its efficacy; in fact, microwaving or steaming makes available even more of this phytochemical.

In tests with mice, phenethyl isothiocyanate (PEITC) has been shown to guard against lung cancer by neutralizing the effects of smoke and other chemicals.

SUPERFOOD SOURCES OF SULFORAPHANE AND OTHER ISOTHIOCYANATES

Broccoli

Brussels sprouts

Cabbage and bok choy

Cauliflower

Collards

Kale

Mustard greens

Turnip, turnip greens, and rutabaga

Watercress

Lignans

Acting as antioxidants, lignans stimulate enzymes that interfere with the action of carcinogens. Because they're found chiefly in flax, they're naturally accompanied by heart-saving omega-3 fatty acids and great fiber. Flaxseed is a new food on the natural foods scene, but well worth finding and adding to home-baked goods.

SUPERFOOD SOURCES OF LIGNANS

Flaxseed, flaxseed oil

Limonene—Effective Anticarcinogen

Potent essence of citrus fruits, limonene increases the production of defensive enzymes that help neutralize carcinogens. In animal trials, limonene has been shown to protect against breast cancer. Researchers in Great Britain have been able to demonstrate not only that limonene works but how it works, and have targeted it for development as a nontoxic breast cancer drug. Limonene is compared to Taxol, a drug derived from the bark of the Pacific yew tree, which is also one of a new class of natural therapeutic drugs. This is not an opportunity for self-medication, however. At present, very high amounts of limonene, which produce unpleasant side effects, are needed to treat cancer, but scientists are hoping to concentrate its efficacy into a smaller dose.

Rich in limonene, citrus fruits also yield a bonus of soluble fiber for the heart and vitamin C for all-around healing.

SUPERFOOD SOURCES OF LIMONENE

Citrus: lemons, oranges, tangerines
  (especially the oil of their rinds)

Phthalides

Well-known denizens of the stew pot, flavorful vegetables and herbs from the feathery-leafed *umbelliferae* family contain phthalides, phytochemicals that inhibit the production of tumors.

SUPERFOOD SOURCES OF PHTHALIDES

Carrots

Celery

Coriander

Dill

Fennel

Parsley

Polyphenols, Including Flavonoids (Bioflavonoids)

Polyphenols are nonnutritional antioxidant compounds that have been credited with protecting the skin from ultraviolet light, improving the cholesterol ratio between the "bad" LDL cholesterol and the "good" HDL cholesterol, lowering blood pressure, protecting the teeth and gums from decay and disease, defending the body against the flu virus, and helping to burn fat—a mighty impressive list of benefits!

Phenolic substances in red wine, but not in white, may be responsible for its antioxidant and blood-thinning properties.

Flavonoids are plant pulp products thought to protect against the bad effects of estrogen and some carcinogens by preventing them from attaching to normal cells. To benefit from flavonoids, which are found in the plant's membranes, you need whole fruits and vegetables rather than juices.

Researchers have found some evidence that flavonoids may reduce the risk of heart disease, but other studies have been far from conclusive. Dietary flavonoids, especially quercetin, however, have been associated with a lower incidence of stroke in a study of over five hundred men who were followed from 1970 to 1985. Flavonoids also flush carcinogens out of the system. So while scientists sort out all the data, it makes sense to enjoy more tea and fruit in the satisfying knowledge that they are contributing to a longer, healthier life.

SUPERFOOD SOURCES OF POLYPHENOLS

Artichokes

Berries: blueberries, strawberries

Fruit and vegetables (pulp and pith), especially citrus, onions, and apples

Red grapes and red wine

SUPERFOOD SOURCES OF FLAVONOIDS

Sweet potatoes

Tea, green and black

Ellagic Acid—Another Cancer-Blocking Phenolic Compound

Found abundantly in fruits and vegetables, ellagic acid detoxifies some well-known carcinogens such as benzopyrene and aflatoxin (which crops up on moldy peanuts and beans). It literally sweeps up free radicals to protect cells from structural damage. In one animal study, a diet high in ellagic acid resulted in over 50 percent fewer esophageal tumors.

Apples
Berries: blackberries, cranberries, strawberries
Grapes
Nuts, especially walnuts

Salicylates—Nature's Aspirin

Aspirin was first discovered as a chemical by-product of the white willow tree, salicin, named for the herb's genus, *Salix*. Belonging to the same family as aspirin, salicylates may behave similarly in helping to prevent blood clotting, and therefore protecting against strokes. Salicylates are found naturally in some plant foods and spices.

SUPERFOOD SOURCES OF SALICYLATES
Herbs and spices: cinnamon, curry, dill, oregano
Oranges
Raspberries
Tomatoes

Saponins

Some of the healthy heart foods contain saponins, substances that lower blood pressure and inhibit cholesterol absorption. Saponins also interfere with DNA replication to help prevent the reproduction of cancer cells.

SUPERFOOD SOURCES OF SAPONINS
Garlic
Herbs
Soybeans and soybean products such as soy milk and tofu

Triterpenoids—Estrogen Suppressors

Some tumor formation is hormone dependent. Triterpenoids inhibit the carcinogenic activity of estrogen, which makes these phytochemicals important in preventing against breast cancer. Their antibacterial properties help to prevent tooth decay and gum disease. Licorice, a prime source of triterpenoids, is known to raise blood pressure, however, and it should be avoided by anyone who has high blood pressure.

SUPERFOOD SOURCES OF TRITERPENOIDS
Citrus fruits
Licorice root
Soybeans and tofu

Protease Inhibitors

Proteases are enzymes that digest protein. Protease inhibitors have been developed by plants to ensure the survival of their species by making their seeds difficult to digest by marauding insects. At first nutritionists believed that protease inhibitors therefore must be antinutritious, but more recent research has found that these enzymes may actually protect humans from cancer by suppressing the malignant process just as they defend plants from species destruction by predators.

SUPERFOOD SOURCES OF PROTEASE
INHIBITORS

Beans, especially soybeans

Eggplant

Potatoes

Rice

Phytoestrogens—Protection Against Problem Hormones

Some foods contain an estrogenlike compound that helps to prevent hormone-related diseases, such as breast and prostate cancers. Although they are a weaker form of the hormone, phytoestrogens bind themselves to receptor sites and thus block the access of more damaging forms of estrogen. Phytoestrogens may also prevent the "see-saw" extremes in fluctuating estrogen levels that are thought to cause menopausal hot flashes.

SUPERFOOD SOURCES OF
PHYTOESTROGENS

Apples

Beans

Beets

Brown rice

Cabbage

Carrots

Citrus fruits

Cornmeal

Fennel

Oatmeal

Potatoes

Radishes

Soybeans and tofu

Whole wheat and whole grains

Genistein—for Whatever Ails You

A class of phytoestrogens, the isoflavones, includes one of special interest called genistein. This compound, found chiefly in soy, seems to act differently in response to different circumstances. It behaves like estrogen in staving off osteoporosis by preventing the resorption of bone. But then it performs as an anti-estrogen in slowing the growth of hormone-related tumors. It helps to control menopausal symptoms, decrease blood cholesterol, and defend against atherosclerosis. Many foods have been called "miracle foods" over the ages, but perhaps none comes closer to deserving that title than soy.

SUPERFOOD SOURCES OF GENISTEIN

Soybeans, soybean products such as soy milk and tofu

Those Colorful Carotenoids

Carotenoids come in several vivid shades, of which the best known is the well-advertised beta-carotene. Following some impressive population studies in which people who ate more green and orange plant foods seemed less at risk for lung cancer and other cancers, scientists hoped they had found a magic bullet in beta-carotene, the most abundant carotenoid. But when they isolated beta-carotene as a supplement and tested it on male smokers in Finland, it flunked—possibly because there are literally hundreds of carotenoids, combined as nature intended in whole foods, that could be responsible for the promise of those early studies. So the best advice is still to eat an abundant variety of carotenoid foods, and thus take advantage of the way they act in concert to protect the body from degenerative diseases. The following palette of carotenoids features those that have been the subject of recent research.

Alpha Carotene—Immunity Builder

This lesser known carotenoid boosts the immune response and peps up overall vitamin A activity. Researchers have found evidence that alpha carotene may defend against lung cancer and some inflammatory disorders.

SUPERFOOD SOURCES OF ALPHA CAROTENE

Carrots
Pumpkin

Beta-carotene—Free-Radical Fighter

A powerful antioxidant, beta-carotene helps to clean up those damaging free radicals that cause us to suffer the effects of aging, from heart disease to cataracts. Beta-carotene works with other antioxidant foods to prevent some forms of cancer. A study in China found that beta-carotene combined with vitamin E and selenium lowered the risk of stomach cancer.

SUPERFOOD SOURCES OF BETA-CAROTENE

Apricots
Cantaloupe
Carrots
Dark green vegetables
Nectarines
Peaches
Pumpkin
Sweet potatoes
Winter squash

Beta Cryptoxanthin—More Insurance for the Lungs

Like alpha carotene, this precursor to vitamin A appears to lessen the risk of lung cancer.

SUPERFOOD SOURCES OF BETA CRYPTOXANTHIN

Mangoes
Oranges
Papayas
Tangerines

Lycopene—Think Red!

Found in red fruits and vegetables, lycopene is a carotenoid closely related to beta-carotene. Harvard researchers have reported that men who eat ten or more servings of lycopene-rich tomatoes and tomato sauce weekly have a 45 percent reduction in the risk of prostate cancer. Even two or three servings have a positive effect—a 34 percent reduction. Cancer risk to the bladder, colon, pancreas, and cervix is also lessened by a diet rich in lycopene.

Recent studies have revealed that older people with below-normal lycopene levels are more liable to need assistance with daily housekeeping and personal tasks and to suffer from mental impairment and depression. As an antioxidant, lycopene is also credited with reducing the risk of heart disease. The most concentrated form of lycopene is probably a rich, thick tomato sauce, which is a good reason never to give up pizza (just make it the low-fat way and add some milled flaxseed to the crust, page 184).

SUPERFOOD SOURCES OF LYCOPENE

Red grapefruit

Tomatoes

Watermelon

Lutein and Zeaxanthin—Think Green!

People whose diets are rich in carotenoids tend to have fewer age-related eye diseases, so for many years the nutritional conclusion was summarized as "eat your carrots." Lately, however, studies have become more finely tuned. Because lutein and zeaxanthin form the yellow pigment in the macula, researchers now theorize that these two carotenoids protect the eyes from macular degeneration. Lutein and zeaxanthin, found in green rather than orange foods, also lessen the risk of several cancers—lung, colon, prostate, and esophageal.

SUPERFOOD SOURCES OF LUTEIN AND ZEAXANTHIN

Broccoli

Chard

Collards

Mustard greens

Okra

Romaine lettuce

Spinach

Turnip greens

Fiber—An Important Nonnutrient

Besides a panoply of vitamins, minerals, and phytochemicals, plant foods also contain an important bonus, *fiber*, which our grandparents called "roughage." Fiber is simply the material from plant cells that is not digested (insoluble fiber) or only partly digested (soluble fiber). These may be skins on corn kernels or peas, seeds on strawberries, filaments in asparagus and broccoli stalks, or the husks on whole grains before they are processed. Fiber is bulky, and that helps to move foods through the intestines more quickly, thus improving the health of the whole digestive system as well as helping to speed any cancer-causing substances out of our systems. Yet the average American consumes only about half the recommended 20 to 30 grams daily. (It's not recommended, however, that a person exceed 35 grams a day, which might speed important vitamins and minerals out of the body or have other adverse effects.)

A diet high in insoluble fiber is the natural way to relieve constipation. Because fiber is like a sponge, it absorbs many times its weight in water, and produces a larger, softer stool that passes easily. This makes it good insurance against the risk of cancers of the colon and rectum as well. Too little fiber can result in diverticulitis, an inflammation of the digestive tract that occurs when waste moves too slowly through the system, or in hemorrhoids, dilated veins caused by straining. These conditions became more common the more foods were refined, as when soft white bread replaced hearty whole-grain bread. Diverticulitis now afflicts one out of three people over the age of fifty.

A recent study in Finland showed that each additional 10 milligrams of fiber that a man consumed reduced his risk of dying from a heart attack by 17 percent. Soluble fibers especially are the heart savers. They're found in oats and barley, in pectin-rich fruits such as apples, and in segmented fruits like grapefruit. Numerous studies have credited this kind of fiber with lowering blood cholesterol. Other research has suggested that soluble fiber may improve control of blood sugar, reducing the need for insulin in some people with diabetes.

You can also benefit from the vitamins, minerals, phytochemicals galore, and lower fat content that go right along with fiber-rich plant foods. This is so true that researchers are not absolutely sure whether it's the fiber or the fiber-plus-nutrients that should take the credit for disease prevention. To those of us who are simply preparing and enjoying good foods, it doesn't really matter. Every food on the high-fiber list is good for us in many other ways; this is what makes them superfoods.

There's more to high fiber than a bowl of bran cereal, which some people simply can't tolerate without suffering from intestinal distress—gas and bloating. If you're one of these sensitive folks, avoid this problem by going slowly as you increase the amount of fiber-rich foods in your diet, always staying in the comfortable range. Don't concentrate on the roughest of "roughage," but enjoy a variety of the fiber-rich foods that follow.

SUPERFOOD SOURCES OF SOLUBLE AND INSOLUBLE FIBER

Apples
Bananas
Barley
Berries
Broccoli
Brown rice
Brussels sprouts
Carrots
Citrus fruits: oranges, tangerines, grapefruit
Corn
Fruits, dried: raisins, prunes
Grains, whole and unrefined, in cereals, bread, and pasta
Legumes: beans and peas
Oats
Potatoes with skins

Water—You Need It More Than You Know

Over half of your body is made up of water, and there isn't a bodily process going on inside you that doesn't require fluids. With ordinary activity, you need to replace 2 to 3 quarts of water a day, but some of that will come from the foods you eat, which are 85 to 95 percent water. The rest you have to drink in the form of soup, juice, or just plain water. If you exercise or the weather is hot, you'll need even more water than thirst will suggest. Thirst can be satisfied before your body's needs are met.

Caffeinated beverages tend to act as diuretics, increasing urine production, so they're not good choices for hydrating the body.

If a funny taste in the tap water or fears about its safety bother you, drink bottled waters instead. They're not healthier in the sense of being more nutritious, but if pouring it from a bottle results in your drinking more water, bottled waters will promote good health.

People who are trying to quit smoking are advised to drink lots of water and other noncaffeinated liquids to flush nicotine out of their bodies faster. Sipping a glass of water can also help to relieve the stress of nicotine withdrawal (at the very least, it's something to keep your mouth and hands busy!).

Ever feel terribly fatigued in the middle of the afternoon? Try a glass of cold water before any other remedy, because fatigue is one sure sign that the body's liquid level has fallen too low. For the same reason, take bottled water with you in the car to fight fatigue while driving.

If plain water seems a bit boring, enliven it with a slice of lemon or lime, or enjoy an occasional bottle of carbonated water sizzling over ice in a stemmed glass. To your very good health!

Beautiful Soups and Stews

Soup is a light, lively way to combine many superfoods in one pot. The best soups are rich in vitamins, minerals, and phytochemicals disguised in a tasty brew. They're often flavored with aromatic root vegetables, abundant in antioxidants and immunity builders, and they're enlivened with members of the feather-leaved, anticancer *umbelliferae* family: celery, fennel, dill, parsley, and cilantro or coriander. Sometimes they're thickened with rice or beans, adding B vitamins and fiber as well.

Whether a soup is considered to be the first course or the main course depends upon the size of the soup bowls (personally, I like large soup *plates* with wide, flat rims) and the substantial nature of the bread served alongside. Or a quick, uncomplicated soup can be a great lunch, the healthy alternative to the ubiquitous ham sandwich.

About stews, however, there is no doubt. These thicker, filling combinations are meant to be the heart of the meal, with perhaps rolls and a salad on the side. Meatless stews, rich in vegetables, beans, and some starchy grain or other, make substantial vegetarian entrees with a "dream team" of ingredients (and complementary amino acids) that supplies complete protein in one dish.

When you or someone for whom you're cooking is stressed or ill, there's nothing more appealing than a clear, fragrant soup with shredded vegetables and comforting small pasta shapes. Beginning with home-made stock or canned broth or even prepared bouillon, a simple, comforting soup, with its nutritional medicine and emotional magic, is culinary "first aid" that can be prepared in less than a half hour. In fact, soup is probably the easiest dish you can make (and most likely was the first made by our remote ancestors, once they tired of grilling).

Asparagus Soup

Rich in heart-helping potassium and folate, this "creamy" soup is an elegant starter.

1 pound asparagus, woody ends removed and cut into 1-inch pieces
1 tablespoon butter
¼ cup chopped shallots
1 tablespoon all-purpose flour
5 cups Chicken-Mushroom Stock (page 333) or canned chicken broth
1 teaspoon chopped fresh thyme or ¼ teaspoon dried
Salt
Freshly ground black pepper
2 teaspoons minced fresh chives
½ cup nonfat plain yogurt, at room temperature

Separate the stalks from asparagus tips. Cook the tips in boiling salted water until just tender, about 3 minutes. Drain and reserve.

In a large saucepan, melt butter and sauté the shallots over medium heat until softened, 3 minutes. Stir in flour and cook, stirring, over very low heat 1 minute. Add the stock, asparagus stalks, thyme, and salt to taste. Simmer the soup, covered, until the asparagus is very tender, 20 minutes.

Remove the asparagus with a slotted spoon and puree it in a food processor, gradually adding about 2 cups of the cooking liquid. Return the pureed mixture to the remaining cooking liquid and whisk to blend. Add pepper to taste. Add the reserved asparagus tips and heat through. Mix the chives with the yogurt. Serve the soup with a dollop of yogurt on each portion.

Makes 4 servings.

Milanese Cabbage and Rice Soup

This delectable soup is just as tasty (but thicker) when warmed up the next day. Lemon gives the broth a unique flavor, and the peel is rich in limonene, an anticancer phytochemical. Cruciferous cabbage itself is a top anticancer vegetable.

2 tablespoons olive oil
1 large yellow onion, chopped
2 garlic cloves, finely chopped
1 pound green or savoy cabbage, coarsely chopped
6 cups chicken or vegetable broth
½ cup Arborio rice or any white rice
4 thin strips of lemon peel (without any white pith)
2 tablespoons fresh lemon juice
  Salt and freshly ground black pepper
  Freshly grated Parmesan cheese, to pass

Heat the oil in a large pot and sauté the onion over medium-high heat until lightly browned, about 5 minutes. Add the garlic during the last minute. Add the cabbage, broth, rice, and lemon peel. Bring the soup to a simmer, cover, and cook 20 minutes. Add the lemon juice. Season with salt and pepper to taste. Pass cheese at the table.

Makes 6 servings.

Kale, Potato, and Carrot Soup
with Balsamic Vinegar

A really quick and easy soup, spiced with black pepper and vinegar instead of sausage.

  1 pound kale, well-washed and coarsely chopped
  8 cups beef stock or broth
  ½ pound peeled baby carrots
  4 potatoes, cut into 2-inch strips
  ¼ teaspoon freshly ground black pepper
  2 to 3 tablespoons balsamic vinegar

Combine the kale and stock in a large pot. Bring mixture to a simmer, cover, and cook 5 minutes. Add the carrots, potatoes, and black pepper. Cover and cook 15 to 20 minutes, until the vegetables are tender. Stir in vinegar to taste.

Makes 6 to 8 servings.

Escarole and Mushroom Soup

This hearty soup can be prepared in less than a half hour—and will receive rave reviews.

  3 tablespoons olive oil
10 ounces mushrooms, preferably brown, cleaned and sliced
 ¼ cup chopped shallots
  1 garlic clove, minced
  1 bunch (about ¾ pound) escarole, well-washed and coarsely chopped
  6 cups Vegetable Stock (page 331), Chicken-Mushroom Stock (page 333), or canned broth
  1 tablespoon chopped fresh basil or ½ teaspoon dried
 ½ teaspoon salt
 ¼ teaspoon freshly ground black pepper
  1 cup tubettini (small pasta tubes)
     Freshly grated Romano cheese, to pass

Heat the oil in a large pot, and sauté the mushrooms over medium heat, stirring often, until mushrooms release their juices, the liquid evaporates, and they begin to brown. Add the shallots and cook, stirring, until nicely colored. Add the garlic and sauté to flavor the oil but not brown it.

Add the escarole, stock, basil, salt, and pepper. Cover and simmer the soup until the escarole is quite tender, 15 to 20 minutes. Meanwhile, cook the tubettini separately according to package directions.

Stir the tubettini into the soup. Pass cheese at the table.

Makes 6 servings.

North African Lentil Soup with Vegetables

There are plenty of immunity-building ingredients in this soup, from garlic and onion to zinc-rich lentils.

1½ cups lentils
 1 tablespoon olive oil
 2 celery stalks, diced
 1 yellow onion, chopped
 2 garlic cloves, minced
 1 tablespoon minced fresh ginger or ½ teaspoon ground ginger
 6 cups water
 3 chicken bouillon cubes (see Note below)
½ teaspoon salt
 1 large carrot, pared and diced
 2 tablespoons tomato paste
½ teaspoon ground cinnamon
 2 cups diced yellow or white potato
½ teaspoon hot pepper sauce or to taste

Pick over and rinse the lentils.

Heat the oil in a large pot over medium heat and sauté the celery, onion, garlic, and fresh ginger until softened and fragrant, about 3 minutes. Add the lentils, water, bouillon cubes, salt, carrot, tomato paste, cinnamon and ground ginger, if using. Bring the soup to a boil. Reduce the heat and simmer, covered, 40 minutes. Add the potato, and continue to simmer, covered, until the lentils and potato are tender, 10 to 15 minutes. Stir in the hot pepper sauce, and keep warm about 3 minutes to blend flavors. Taste and correct seasoning, if needed.

Makes 6 servings.

NOTE

Some bouillon cubes make 2 cups broth; some make 1 cup. Read the package directions and adjust the amount needed for 6 cups.

Curried Chick-pea Soup with Butternut Squash and Greens

Antioxidants abound in this flavorful soup.

- 2 tablespoons olive oil
- 1 red bell pepper, seeded and diced
- 1 large yellow onion, chopped
- 1 garlic clove, minced
- 2 teaspoons mild or spicy curry powder
- 6 cups Vegetable Stock (page 331), Chicken-Mushroom Stock (page 333), or canned broth
  About ¾ pound butternut squash, peeled and cubed
- 2 cups finely chopped greens, such as fresh spinach, collards, or chard
- 2 cups cooked chick-peas (page 328) or 1 (14- to 15-oz.) can, drained and rinsed
  Salt and freshly ground black pepper (optional)

Heat the oil in a large pot over medium heat and sauté the bell pepper, onion, and garlic until sizzling and fragrant. Stir in the curry powder. Blend in the stock and bring to a boil. Add the squash, greens, and chick-peas. Bring the soup back to a boil, reduce heat, and simmer until squash is tender, 15 to 20 minutes. Taste before adding salt and pepper; the soup is quite flavorful without them.

Makes 6 servings.

Tomato-Yogurt Soup with Fresh Dill

A chilled soup that's perfect for a summer luncheon. Nonfat yogurt is a healthy way to boost calcium.

2 tablespoons olive oil
4 shallots, chopped
4 cups fresh, very ripe tomatoes, peeled, seeded, and chopped (see Note below)
2 cups Chicken-Mushroom Stock (page 333) or canned broth
1 teaspoon sugar
½ teaspoon celery salt
⅛ teaspoon white pepper
1 cup plain nonfat yogurt
¼ cup loosely packed chopped fresh dill
   Paper-thin slices of unpeeled cucumber and fresh dill sprigs, for garnish

Heat the oil in a large saucepan over medium heat and sauté the shallots until soft and fragrant, about 3 minutes. Add the tomatoes, stock, sugar, celery salt, and pepper, and bring to a boil. Reduce the heat, cover, and simmer the soup 15 minutes. Allow it to cool to room temperature.

Puree the soup in 2 batches in a blender or food processor, adding ½ cup yogurt to each. Combine the batches in a bowl and stir in the chopped dill. Cover and chill the soup. Serve the soup cold, garnished with cucumber slices and dill sprigs.

Makes 6 servings.

NOTE
Substitute 1 (28-oz.) can tomatoes in juice, not puree, for fresh tomatoes. If you use canned tomatoes, reduce the stock to 1½ cups.

Italian Farmer's Soup with Sage

Once upon a time, before preservatives, two-day-old bread used to become stale, so thrifty farm folk invented this savory soup.

¼ cup olive oil
4 garlic cloves, minced
4 cups roughly cubed Italian bread (small cubes)
4 cups peeled, seeded, and chopped fresh ripe tomatoes
4 cups vegetable or chicken broth
½ teaspoon salt
⅛ teaspoon hot red pepper flakes
⅛ teaspoon freshly ground black pepper
2 tablespoons minced fresh flat-leaf parsley
8 fresh sage leaves, minced

Heat the oil in a large pot over medium heat and sauté the garlic until it sizzles. Add the bread and cook, stirring, until it's lightly colored, 3 to 5 minutes. Add all the remaining ingredients except the herbs, and bring to a boil. Reduce the heat and simmer the soup, covered, 20 minutes. Stir in the herbs during the last few minutes of cooking. Let the soup stand off the heat 5 minutes before serving.

Makes 6 servings.

Glory-of-Summer Gazpacho with Parsley Pesto

A favorite cold soup that's equally at home in a formal setting or on a picnic.

1   garlic clove, peeled and halved
1   slice whole-wheat bread with crusts, torn into pieces
3   cups very ripe, peeled, seeded, chopped tomatoes (about 4)
1   cucumber, peeled, seeded, and chopped
1   green bell pepper, seeded and chopped
4   scallions, chopped
    About 1 cup tomato juice
3   tablespoons wine vinegar
3   tablespoons olive oil
½   teaspoon salt
¼   teaspoon hot pepper sauce
    A few dashes Worcestershire sauce
¼   cup Parsley-Walnut Pesto (page 327)

With the motor running, toss the garlic down the feed tube of a food processor to mince it. Add the bread pieces and process into crumbs. Stop the motor, add the vegetables, and pulse the vegetables and bread until very finely chopped. Transfer to a bowl and stir in 1 cup tomato juice, vinegar, oil, salt, hot pepper sauce, and Worcestershire sauce. Add more tomato juice if needed to create a thick soup texture. Cover and chill the soup.

When ready to serve, garnish each serving with a swirl of pesto.
Makes 4 servings.

Vegetarian Vegetable Soup

No need for stock or broth in this soup; it makes its own broth, and very tasty it is, too!

2 to 3 tablespoons olive oil
6 ounces mushrooms, cleaned and sliced
2 or 3 leeks, well washed and chopped
1 cup diced celery or fennel bulb
2 garlic cloves, minced
3 cups peeled, seeded, chopped fresh tomatoes or 1 (28-oz.) can imported Italian tomatoes with juice
2 cups diced potato
2 large carrots, pared and thinly sliced on diagonal
2 cups shredded savoy or green cabbage
1 bay leaf
5 cups water
½ pound fresh green beans, trimmed and cut into 1-inch pieces
1 small zucchini or summer squash, cut into 1-inch chunks
2 teaspoons chopped fresh thyme or ½ teaspoon dried
¾ teaspoon salt or to taste
¼ teaspoon ground black pepper

Heat 2 tablespoons oil in a large nonstick pot over medium heat, and sauté the mushrooms, stirring often, until their juice evaporates and they brown. Add more oil only if needed. Add the leeks and celery, and sauté, stirring, until vegetables are softened, 5 minutes. Add the garlic and cook 1 minute longer.

Add the tomatoes, potato, carrots, cabbage, bay leaf, and water. Bring to a simmer, cover, and cook 20 minutes. Add the green beans, zucchini, thyme, salt, and pepper. Simmer until all the vegetables are tender, about 10 minutes. Remove the bay leaf before serving. Taste and correct seasoning; add more salt, if desired.

Makes 6 servings.

Vegetable Soup, Mexican Style

Canola oil is high in monounsaturated fatty acids, good for reducing "bad" (LDL) cholesterol.

2   tablespoons canola oil
2   mild green chiles, seeded and chopped
1   large yellow onion, chopped
2   celery stalks with leaves, chopped
1   garlic clove, finely chopped
6   cups Vegetable Stock (page 331), Chicken-Mushroom Stock (page 333), or canned broth
1   (15-to 16-oz.) can tomatoes with juice
2   teaspoons chopped fresh cilantro or ½ teaspoon dried
2   teaspoons chopped fresh basil or ½ teaspoon dried
½   teaspoon salt
⅛   teaspoon freshly ground pepper or to taste
2   large carrots, pared and thinly sliced on diagonal into 1-inch slices
1   cup canned chick-peas, drained and rinsed, or 1 cup cooked (page 328)
1   medium zucchini, quartered lengthwise and cut into 1-inch pieces
1   cup fresh shelled or frozen green peas
1   small ripe avocado, for garnish

Heat the oil in a large pot over low heat and slowly "sweat" the chiles, onion, celery, and garlic, uncovered, until soft but not brown, about 10 minutes. Add the stock, tomatoes, cilantro, basil, salt, pepper, carrots, and chick-peas. Cover and simmer 15 minutes. Add the zucchini and peas. Simmer 10 minutes or until vegetables are tender. Pit, peel and slice avocado; garnish soup just before serving.

Makes 6 servings.

September Vegetable Chowder

A meal in itself, featuring the vegetables of late summer in the northern regions of the country: The corn is still great, the late tomatoes are bursting with goodness, and the zucchinis are coming in big, especially from home gardens.

2   tablespoons olive oil
2   leeks, well-washed and chopped
1   cup chopped celery
1   red bell pepper, seeded and cut into triangles
1   mild green chile, seeded and chopped
2   cups peeled, seeded, and chopped tomatoes
2   large red boiling potatoes, peeled or unpeeled, cut into 1-inch chunks
4   cups Vegetable Stock (page 331), Chicken-Mushroom Stock (page 333), or canned broth
2   cups fresh corn kernels
1   large zucchini, cut into 1-inch chunks
½   teaspoon salt
⅛   teaspoon freshly ground pepper
¼   cup nonfat dry milk
2   tablespoons cornstarch
1   cup milk
2   tablespoons chopped fresh flat-leaf parsley
1   tablespoon chopped fresh basil
    Rye bread (optional)

Heat the oil in a large pot over medium heat and sauté the leeks, celery, bell pepper, and chile until they are softened, about 10 minutes. Add the tomatoes, potatoes, and stock; cover and simmer 10 minutes. Add the corn, zucchini, salt, and pepper; cover and simmer 8 to 10 minutes or until all vegetables are tender.

Whisk the dry milk and cornstarch into the liquid milk and add it to the simmering chowder. Cook, stirring constantly, until the mixture bubbles and thickens slightly. Stir in the parsley and basil. Serve in bowls with fresh rye bread on the side, if desired.

Makes 4 servings.

Gingery Shrimp, Carrot, and Scallion Soup

For quick soups, pastas, and stir-fries, a large bag of good-quality cooked, cleaned shrimp in the freezer is a great time-saver.

1   tablespoon olive oil
½   pound carrots, diced
1   bunch scallions, chopped
1   small red bell pepper, seeded and diced
2   slices fresh ginger, minced
7   cups Vegetable Stock (page 331), Chicken-Mushroom Stock (page 333), or canned broth
½   cup orzo (rice-shaped pasta)
½   pound cooked, peeled, cleaned small shrimp
2   tablespoons minced fresh cilantro or flat-leaf parsley
¼   teaspoon Spicy Mixed Pepper (page 335) or white pepper

Heat the oil in a large pot over medium heat and sauté the carrots, scallions, bell pepper, and ginger until sizzling. Add the stock and simmer until the vegetables are tender, 10 minutes.

Cook and drain the orzo according to package directions. Stir the cooked orzo, shrimp, cilantro or parsley, and mixed pepper into the soup. Bring to a simmer and immediately remove from the heat. Let stand 3 minutes before serving.

Makes 6 servings.

Scallop, Chard, and Sweet Potato Stew

This is a main-dish soup you can have ready in twenty minutes. A sliced tomato and cucumber salad and crusty rye bread could complete the menu.

    2 tablespoons olive oil
    ¼ cup chopped shallots
    1 large (about ¾ pound) sweet potato, diced
    1 bunch chard (½ pound) or escarole, well-washed and chopped
       coarsely into 2-inch pieces
    6 cups Vegetable Stock (page 331), Chicken-Mushroom Stock
       (page 333), or canned broth
    4 strips lemon peel (with no white pith)
    1 teaspoon chopped fresh thyme or ¼ teaspoon dried
    ½ teaspoon salt (optional)
    1 pound bay scallops, rinsed
    1 cup orecchiette (ear-shaped pasta)
       Freshly ground black pepper

Heat the oil in a large pot over medium heat and sauté the shallots until they are lightly colored, about 3 minutes. Add the sweet potato, chard, stock, lemon peel, and thyme, and bring to a boil. Reduce the heat, cover, and simmer until the vegetables are tender, 10 to 15 minutes. Taste the broth, adding salt if necessary.

Stir in the scallops and simmer until they are cooked through, 3 to 5 minutes. Meanwhile, cook and drain the pasta according to package directions. Stir the pasta and pepper to your taste into the soup. If possible, serve the stew in old-fashioned wide soup plates.

Makes 4 servings.

Scallop and Clam Soup with Fennel

A variation on a traditional soup of Provence.

 2 tablespoons olive oil
 1 small yellow onion, chopped
 1 small red bell pepper, seeded and diced
 1 cup chopped fennel
 1 large garlic clove, minced
 1 cup peeled, seeded, and chopped fresh tomatoes, or canned
    tomatoes, undrained
 2 cups [2 (8-oz.) bottles] clam juice
 3 cups Vegetable Stock (page 331) or canned broth
 ¾ to 1 pound (2 large) boiling potatoes, peeled and diced
 1 tablespoon chopped fresh flat-leaf parsley
 1 teaspoon chopped fresh thyme or ¼ teaspoon dried
 1 bay leaf
 ½ teaspoon salt
 ¼ teaspoon freshly ground black pepper
 ¼ teaspoon saffron threads, crushed between the fingers
 ¾ pound bay scallops, rinsed
 ½ pound chopped fresh clams
    Crusty bread

Heat the oil in a large pot over medium heat and sauté the onion, bell pepper, and fennel until they are lightly colored, about 8 minutes. Add the garlic during the last minute. Add the tomatoes and sauté 10 minutes. Add the clam juice, stock, potatoes, parsley, thyme, bay leaf, salt, pepper, and saffron. Bring to a simmer, cover, and cook until potatoes are tender, about 15 minutes.

Add the scallops and clams and simmer 5 minutes longer. Remove the bay leaf. Serve with a bakery-fresh crusty bread.

Makes 6 servings.

New England Scallop and Fish Chowder

A lighter and easier version of the creamy original. Traditionally, this chowder would be served with common crackers or pilot crackers.

2 tablespoons canola oil
1 large onion, chopped
1 (8-oz.) bottle clam juice
1 pound potatoes, peeled and cut into 1-inch wedges
½ teaspoon salt
¼ cup nonfat dry milk
3 tablespoons instant flour, such as Wondra
3 cups milk
¾ pound bay scallops, rinsed
½ to ¾ pound fresh haddock fillet (or any white fish),
   cut into 1-inch chunks
1 teaspoon chopped fresh thyme
¼ teaspoon white pepper
⅛ teaspoon cayenne pepper

Heat the oil in a large pot over medium heat and sauté the onion until soft, 3 to 5 minutes. Add the clam juice, potatoes, and salt. Bring to a boil and cook until the potatoes are tender, about 15 minutes. Partially mash the potatoes, leaving some larger chunks.

Whisk the dry milk and flour into the liquid milk, and add mixture to the pot. Bring to a boil over medium heat, stirring constantly, and cook until bubbling and slightly thickened. Add the scallops, haddock, thyme, white pepper, and cayenne. Simmer, stirring often, until the scallops and fish are opaque, 3 to 5 minutes. Let stand off heat 5 minutes to blend flavors.

Makes 4 servings as a main dish, 6 as a first course.

Chicken, Butternut, and White Bean Stew

As stews go, this is one of the quickest cooking because it uses boned chicken instead of beef. Serve with a nice cool salad of mixed dark greens, and dinner is complete!

- 1   pound boneless, skinless chicken breasts, cut into 1-inch chunks
- ¼   cup all-purpose flour
-     About 2 tablespoons olive oil
- 1   medium yellow onion, chopped
- 1   celery stalk with leaves, chopped
- 1   (15- to 16-oz.) can imported Italian plum tomatoes with juice
- 2   cups Chicken-Mushroom Stock (page 333) or canned broth
- 1   teaspoon chopped fresh oregano or ¼ teaspoon dried
- 1   teaspoon chopped fresh rosemary or ¼ teaspoon dried
- ½   teaspoon salt
- ¼   teaspoon pepper
- 2 to 2½ cups 1-inch butternut squash chunks
- 1   (14- to 16-oz.) can white kidney beans (cannellini), drained and rinsed, or 2 cups cooked (page 328)

Put the flour into a plastic bag with the chicken. Holding the bag closed, shake it to coat the chicken with flour. Shake off excess flour; set chicken aside.

Heat the olive oil in a Dutch oven over low heat and slowly sauté the onion and celery until soft, 3 to 5 minutes. Remove the onion and celery with a slotted spoon; reserve.

Increase heat to medium-high and cook the chicken until browned, adding more oil if needed. Return the vegetables to the pot. Add the tomatoes, stock, oregano, rosemary, salt, pepper, and squash. Break up the tomatoes with a cooking spoon. Bring to a simmer, cover, and cook, stirring occasionally, until the squash is tender and the chicken is cooked through, 20 to 25 minutes. Add the beans, bring back to a simmer, and cook, uncovered, over very low heat about 10 minutes to develop the flavor.

Makes 4 servings.

Beef and Root Vegetable Stew with Polenta

Vegetables predominate in this light beef stew, a New England–style dish that teams up very comfortably with Italian polenta.

¾ pound stewing beef, well-trimmed and cut into small pieces, about ¾ inch
¼ cup all-purpose flour
2 tablespoons olive oil
5 ounces mushrooms, cleaned and sliced
1 garlic clove, chopped
1 red bell pepper, seeded and diced
2 cups pared baby carrots, halved
1½ cups peeled and diced rutabaga
2 medium yellow onions, quartered
2 cups water
1 beef bouillon cube
1 teaspoon sweet paprika
¼ teaspoon dried thyme
½ teaspoon salt
  Freshly ground black pepper
  About 3½ cups hot Make-It-Easy Polenta (page 326)

Combine the meat and flour in a plastic bag. Hold the bag closed and shake it to coat the meat. Shake off excess flour; set meat aside.

Heat 1 tablespoon of the oil in a Dutch oven or large heavy pot over medium-high heat and stir-fry the mushrooms until they release their juices and begin to brown. Remove the mushrooms; reserve. Add the remaining 1 tablespoon of oil and brown the meat. Reduce the heat to medium, add garlic and bell pepper, and sauté until they are softened, about 3 minutes.

Return the mushrooms to the pot. Add the carrots, rutabaga, and onions. Add the water, bouillon cube, paprika, thyme, and salt, scraping the bottom of the pot with a wooden spoon to loosen the brown bits. Bring the stew to a simmer, cover, and cook until the meat is quite tender, 45 minutes to 1 hour. The flour on the meat will thicken the stew. If the stew gets too thick, add a little water. Add pepper to your taste.

Serve the stew with a mound of hot polenta on the side.
Makes 4 servings.

Heart and Sole—Why Seafood Is a Super Dish

One of the heart-healthiest of protein foods, seafood in general has less cholesterol and less fat than lean meat. The fat it does contain is rich in the omega-3 fatty acids that give fish its well-documented reputation as a heart saver. The omega-3s defend against arteriosclerosis and help to prevent strokes. In animal studies, arrhythmia (irregular heartbeats that can trigger sudden death) was reduced when the diet was enriched with the omega-3s, so fish also protects heart rhythm. And you don't have to gorge on fish to benefit. Recent research has concluded that simply dining on fish a couple of times a week is as effective as six weekly helpings.

Shellfish has more cholesterol than other seafood, but it's a cholesterol that seems to be less well absorbed than, say, the cholesterol in eggs. In one study, the cholesterol in a shrimp diet (and shrimp is the seafood highest in cholesterol even among shellfish) raised the "good" HDL blood cholesterol but not the "bad" LDL cholesterol, whereas an egg diet raised both.

The benefits of the omega-3s extend far beyond the cardiovascular system. By suppressing the formation of hormonelike agents called prostaglandins, the omega-3s exert an influence on the immune response and inflammation that may slow the progress of rheumatoid arthritis or even lower the risk of developing the disease in the first place.

Glucose intolerance is significantly lower in people who eat fish than in nonfish eaters. The results of research into this diet connection suggest that a small amount of fish may protect older adults against the development of glucose intolerance and diabetes mellitus.

Is fish also good brain food? What we do know is that the omega-3s enhance early brain and retinal development, which is why pregnant women are urged to include plenty of seafood in their diets.

The protein power of fish is important, too. Studies show that some people over the age of fifty-five are not getting enough protein, and less protein means less energy and a compromised immune system. Speaking of energy, a light (low in fat) protein lunch is a real brain energizer as well. Protein eaten without fat boosts the amino acid tyrosine, which in turn stimulates your brain to produce more of the neurotransmitters dopamine and norepinephrine. The result is a more quick-witted, alert, and confident you.

There's no doubt that any kind of fish is a longevity food, but the so-called "fatty fish" offer the most omega-3 fatty acids (page 32). As a bonus to the cook, there are lots of varieties from which to choose, and cooking every one of them is a cinch. Fish "steaks" can be broiled or baked in a hot oven in just a few minutes, and shellfish steamed in even less time—*fast food* and *home cooking* are not contradictory terms when you're dining on seafood!

Swordfish with Rosemary and "Chips"

Everyone loves potatoes "oven-fried" this way, and fortunately, very little oil is needed to achieve a nice crispy crust!

  3 russet potatoes, peeled
  1 tablespoon olive oil
      Salt and freshly ground black pepper
  1 (1¼- to 1½-lb.) swordfish steak (about 1 inch thick)
  ½ cup seasoned bread crumbs
  ¼ teaspoon grated lemon peel
  2 teaspoons finely chopped fresh rosemary or ½ teaspoon dried
      Lemon wedges

Preheat the oven to 400F (205C).

Cut each potato in half lengthwise, then cut each half lengthwise into 3 pieces the size of fat french fries. Put them into a large baking dish (one that will hold both potatoes and fish in one layer) from which you can serve. Add the oil and stir to coat the potatoes on all sides. Season the potatoes with salt and pepper. Bake them for 15 to 20 minutes, until they're about half-cooked. Remove from the oven, loosen them gently to keep the crispy crust intact, and push them to the sides of the pan.

Rinse and drain the swordfish. Mix together the crumbs and the grated peel. Top the swordfish with the crumbs and arrange it the middle of the pan. Sprinkle everything with the rosemary.

Bake on the top shelf until the fish flakes at the center when tested with a fork and the potatoes are crisp and tender, about 20 minutes. Serve with lemon wedges.

Makes 4 servings.

Poached Salmon and Asparagus in Lettuce Leaves with Cucumber Raita

Easy elegance: The coolness of the raita complements the robust flavor of the salmon.

  Raita (see below)
4 (about 4-oz. each) salmon fillets
12 asparagus spears
10 to 12 outer leaves of a head of romaine lettuce, washed and cut in half crosswise
1 cup hot Vegetable Stock (page 331) or canned broth

Raita
1 cup nonfat plain yogurt
1 cucumber, seeded and finely diced
1 tablespoon chopped fresh chives
¼ teaspoon white pepper

Preheat the oven to 325F (165C).

Prepare Raita: Blend all ingredients together in a small bowl. Cover and chill the raita while cooking the salmon.

Rinse the salmon fillets. Rinse the asparagus and remove the tough ends.

Line a large (13 × 9-inch) oven-to-table baking dish with half of the leaves of romaine lettuce, overlapping. Arrange the fillets over the lettuce, and place the asparagus spears between and around them. Cover with the remaining lettuce leaves. Pour the broth over all.

Lay a sheet of foil loosely over the pan, not touching the lettuce. Poach in the oven until the fish flakes at the center when tested with a fork, about 25 minutes.

To serve, remove the top layer of lettuce. Pass the raita as an accompaniment.

Makes 4 servings.

Fresh Salmon Cakes with Mango

Add steamed new potatoes and a dish of fresh peas, perhaps with summer squash and mint, to create a new-twist-on-tradition Fourth-of-July menu.

2 (6- to 8-oz. each) fresh salmon fillets
   Sprigs of fresh dill
½ cup dry white wine or bottled clam juice
2 cups fresh bread crumbs (from 2 slices bread)
2 tablespoons chopped fresh chives
1 large egg, beaten, or ¼ cup egg substitute
   Salt and freshly ground black pepper to taste
1 tablespoon cornmeal
   About 2 tablespoons olive oil
1 large ripe mango, peeled and sliced

Rinse and pat dry the fillets. Place them in a skillet and lay the dill sprigs over them. Pour in the wine. Poach the fillets, covered, at a very gentle simmer until the salmon flakes at the center when tested with a fork, 8 to 10 minutes. Cool slightly. Discard the skin, if any, and chop the fish coarsely. You should have about 2 cups.

Mix the salmon, crumbs, chives, egg, salt, and pepper. Using about ¼ cup for each, form the mixture into 8 cakes. Lay the cakes on a plate and flatten them slightly. Sprinkle with half the cornmeal. Turn the cakes and sprinkle the other side with the remaining cornmeal. Cover and chill.

Coat a 12-inch skillet with 1 tablespoon of the oil, and fry the cakes over medium heat until they are brown on both sides, turning and adding more oil, if needed. Remove the cakes and keep them warm. Add the mango slices to the pan and heat just long enough to warm them slightly.

Divide the cakes and mango among 4 plates and serve.
Makes 4 servings.

Salmon Mousse

This makes an attractive luncheon dish or addition to an appetizer buffet.

¾ cup clam juice or prepared fish bouillon
1 package unflavored gelatin
1 cup cooked fresh salmon or 1 (7- to 8-oz.) can pink salmon, drained
1 medium potato, cooked, peeled, and chopped (¾ cup cubes)
1 tablespoon rice vinegar
½ teaspoon dried dill weed
½ teaspoon celery salt
¼ teaspoon dry mustard
¼ teaspoon white pepper
½ cup nonfat plain yogurt
1 tablespoon drained capers
1 tablespoon chopped fresh chives
½ cup chopped sweet onion, for garnish
1 cup dill pickle slices, for garnish
4 hard-cooked eggs, peeled and sliced, for garnish (optional)
   Cocktail rye bread

Pour the clam juice into a small saucepan and sprinkle with the gelatin. Let stand 5 minutes to soften. Heat, stirring, until the gelatin is completely dissolved. Cool slightly.

In a food processor, puree the salmon and potato. Add the vinegar, dill, celery salt, mustard, and pepper, and pulse to combine. Add gelatin mixture and pulse to combine. Transfer mixture to a bowl and whisk in the yogurt, capers, and chives.

Spray a 3-cup fish mold or any mold with nonstick baking spray. Pour the mousse into the mold and smooth the top. Cover with plastic wrap and chill overnight.

To unmold, dip mold in warm water up to rim for a few seconds. Place a platter on top and carefully invert. Garnish by surrounding the mousse with chopped onion, dill pickles, and sliced hard-boiled eggs, if desired. Serve with rye bread.

Makes about 3 cups.

Baked Sole with Portobello Mushroom Stuffing

Easily doubled or tripled (using a larger gratin pan), these roll-ups are a pleasing buffet dish.

2 tablespoons olive oil
6 ounces Portobello mushrooms, cleaned and diced
1 cup fresh bread crumbs (from 1 slice white bread)
½ teaspoon dried tarragon
¼ teaspoon dried oregano
¼ teaspoon salt
⅛ teaspoon pepper
   About 1 tablespoon dry white wine, broth, or water
8 sole fillets (about 1½ lbs. total)
4 scallions, chopped
2 tablespoons mayonnaise
½ cup crushed cracker crumbs
   Paprika

Make the stuffing: Heat 1½ tablespoons of the oil in a large nonstick skillet over medium heat and sauté the mushrooms, stirring often, until their juices evaporate and they brown. Stir in the bread crumbs, tarragon, oregano, salt, and pepper. Add enough wine to moisten the stuffing.

Preheat the oven to 400F (205C). Rinse and pat dry the fillets.

Pour the remaining ½ tablespoon of oil into a medium gratin pan, and sprinkle it with the scallions. Divide the stuffing among the fillets, and roll them up. If necessary, use wooden picks to secure the rolls. Place them, seam sides down, in the prepared pan. Spread a little mayonnaise on each. Sprinkle them with cracker crumbs and paprika.

Bake in the top third of the oven 15 to 20 minutes, until the fish flakes at the center when tested with a fork. If you've used wooden picks, remove them before serving.

Makes 4 servings.

Oven-fried Fillets of Sole Amandine

Egg substitute makes a fine low-fat coating for fish and other "fried" foods. It has the advantage of being easy to measure, and contains no cholesterol.

 4 sole fillets, each about 6 ounces
 ¼ cup unbleached all-purpose flour
    About ⅓ cup egg substitute
 ¼ cup seasoned dry bread crumbs
 ¼ cup fine cornmeal
 ½ teaspoon salt
 ⅛ teaspoon freshly ground pepper
 4 scallions, chopped
 1 tablespoon butter
 ½ cup blanched, slivered almonds
 3 tablespoons dry vermouth or dry white wine
 2 tablespoons fresh lemon juice
 1 tablespoon minced fresh flat-leaf parsley

Rinse the fish and pat dry with paper towels. Put the flour on a sheet of waxed paper. Pour the egg substitute into a shallow bowl. On a second sheet of waxed paper, mix the bread crumbs, cornmeal, salt, and pepper. Using two forks, dust each fillet with flour, then dip it in egg substitute, and finally in the crumb mixture to form an even coating on both sides. Arrange in one layer on a plate and chill the fish to set the coating, about 30 minutes.

Preheat the oven to 450F (230C). Oil a large baking dish that will hold the fish in one layer, and scatter the scallions over the bottom. Arrange the fish in the pan in one layer and bake until golden, 15 to 20 minutes. Transfer the fish to a platter and keep it warm.

In a small skillet, melt the butter over medium heat and sauté the almonds until they are lightly colored, about 5 minutes. Stir in the vermouth and lemon juice. Heat, stirring, until the sauce bubbles. Spoon the sauce over the sole, and sprinkle with the parsley.

Makes 4 servings.

Tuna with Peas and Parsleyed New Potatoes

As a quick-company entree, this dish takes less than a half hour to prepare and looks beautiful on a serving plate.

1½ pounds tuna steaks, cut into 1-inch-thick slices
   About ½ cup all-purpose flour for coating
2 tablespoons olive oil, plus more if needed
1 celery stalk, finely diced
1 small yellow onion, finely diced
1 large garlic clove, minced
1½ cups fresh shelled or 1 (10-oz.) package frozen green peas, thawed to separate
2 tablespoons tomato paste
¾ cup hot water
¼ teaspoon salt
   Freshly ground black pepper
   Hot pepper sauce (optional)
   About 20 small whole unpeeled new potatoes, well scrubbed, or 5 large red potatoes, quartered
1 tablespoon chopped fresh flat-leaf parsley
1 tablespoon chopped fresh chives or 1 teaspoon dried chives

Rinse the tuna and pat dry. Remove any skin or very dark red muscle meat. Coat the tuna with flour, shaking off the excess. Heat the oil in a 12-inch skillet over medium-high heat and fry the tuna until lightly browned and cooked through, about 7 minutes. Remove the tuna; set aside.

Add the celery, onion, and garlic, and slowly sauté until lightly colored, 5 minutes, adding more oil, if needed. Add the peas, tomato paste, water, salt, and pepper. Cover and simmer until the peas are tender, 5 to 8 minutes. Return the tuna to the pan and heat through. If desired, add a few dashes of hot pepper sauce.

Meanwhile, steam the potatoes until tender, 10 to 15 minutes. Toss them with the parsley and chives. Spoon the tuna and peas onto a platter and surround them with the potatoes.

Makes 4 servings.

Seared Fresh Tuna Salad with Oranges and Artichoke Hearts

The sweet-tart orange flavor complements the rich taste of tuna. Serve with a crusty white bread on the side.

  4 (5- to 6-oz. each) fresh tuna or swordfish steaks
  ½ teaspoon dried oregano
  ¼ teaspoon salt
  ⅛ teaspoon freshly ground pepper
     Canola oil
  2 seedless oranges, peel and pith removed, segmented
  1 (14-oz.) can artichoke hearts, drained, rinsed, and halved
  2 tablespoons extra-virgin olive oil
  1 tablespoon chopped fresh flat-leaf parsley, plus additional sprigs
     for garnish

  Rinse the fish and pat dry. Remove any skin or very dark red muscle meat. Combine the oregano, salt, and pepper, and rub it into both sides of the fish. Heat a heavy nonstick or cast-iron frying pan over high heat, adding just enough canola oil to coat the bottom. When the pan is quite hot, sear the steaks, two at a time, on both sides. Reduce the heat to medium, cover, and continue cooking until the fish is just cooked through, about 4 minutes more. Do not overcook; the centers should be moist.

  Allow the fish to cool until it's just warm. Divide the steaks among 4 plates. Arrange the orange segments and artichoke hearts on top. Dress each serving with ½ tablespoon olive oil and a little chopped parsley. Garnish the salads with parsley sprigs.

  Makes 4 servings.

Tuna and Chopped Vegetable Salad

Made in a jiffy in the food processor, this tuna salad is both lighter and more nutritious than the usual ones. It makes a fresh-tasting sandwich filling for either pita bread pockets or caraway light rye bread.

1 large carrot, scraped and cut into 4 pieces
2 scallions, cut into 4 pieces
2 celery stalks with leaves, cut into 4 pieces
2 sprigs of fresh parsley, cut into 2 pieces
1 (7- to 8-oz.) can water-packed white tuna, drained
2 tablespoons nonfat plain yogurt
1 tablespoon mayonnaise
  Several dashes black and cayenne peppers

Chop the carrot in a food processor into a very small dice. Add the scallions, celery, and parsley. Pulse to chop (they chop more quickly than the carrot). Add the tuna, yogurt, mayonnaise, and peppers. Pulse until just blended but with some texture; do not overprocess into a mush.

Makes enough filling for 4 sandwiches.

Scrod with Sweet Potatoes and Roasted Bell Peppers

This attractive all-in-one main dish is especially rich in carotenes. Just add a cool salad of mixed greens.

  2 red bell peppers (see Note, opposite)
     Salt and freshly ground black pepper
  2 large sweet potatoes, peeled and sliced crosswise into ½-inch-thick rounds
1½ pounds scrod (preferably in 1 large piece)
  2 tablespoons olive oil
  ½ cup chopped shallots
  1 cup fresh bread crumbs
  1 teaspoon chopped fresh rosemary or ¼ teaspoon dried
     Paprika

Preheat broiler. Roast the peppers about 4 inches below heat source, turning them as they brown, until they are blistered and tender. Remove them to a covered casserole dish. When the peppers are cool enough to handle, slip off the skins; seed and core them. Cut them into strips; season them with salt and pepper to taste.

Parboil the potatoes in boiling salted water until just tender, about 5 minutes. Drain well.

Preheat the oven to 400F (205C). Rinse the fish and pat dry on paper towels.

Put the oil and shallots into a baking pan that will fit the fish with 1 inch to spare all around. Heat the shallots in the oven until they begin to sizzle, about 5 minutes.

Remove pan from the oven. Scoop out and reserve about half the oil and shallots. Lay the potato slices over the remaining shallots. Salt and pepper them, if desired. Reserve a few bell pepper strips, and arrange the rest over the potatoes. Lay the scrod over the vegetables. Brush with the reserved shallots and oil. Sprinkle with the bread crumbs, rosemary, and a few dashes of paprika. Garnish with reserved bell pepper strips. Bake in the top third of the oven until the fish flakes easily at the center, about 20 minutes.

Makes 4 servings.

NOTE

In a hurry? Use roasted bell peppers from a jar.

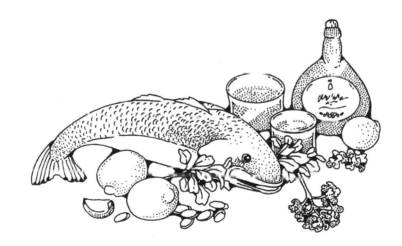

Baked Scrod with Roasted Broccoli

Broccoli and seafood together make a super-healthful dinner. A side dish of tomato salad would round it out to perfection.

    1 pound trimmed fresh broccoli spears
    1 cup herb stuffing mix
    2 tablespoons freshly grated Parmesan cheese
    ½ teaspoon dried tarragon
1½ pounds scrod fillets
       Cayenne pepper
       Lemon wedges

Preheat the oven to 400F (205C).

Cut the broccoli spears lengthwise into stalks that are about ½ inch thick. Parboil them in boiling salted water about 2 minutes after the water returns to a boil. Drain.

Put stuffing mix into a food processor and process until reduced to large crumbs. Add the cheese and tarragon and pulse to combine.

Rinse and pat dry the scrod. Lay the broccoli stalks, stems toward the center, in a large baking dish from which you can serve. Lay the scrod across the stalks. Season the fish with cayenne to taste. Sprinkle with the stuffing mixture.

Bake 15 to 20 minutes, until the fish flakes at the center when tested with a fork. Serve with lemon wedges.

Makes 4 servings.

Scrod with Lemon Sauce

A creamy, comforting fish dish.

1½ pounds scrod
  1 cup low-fat milk
  2 tablespoons nonfat dry milk
  2 tablespoons instant flour, such as Wondra
  ¼ teaspoon dried thyme
  ¼ teaspoon celery salt
  ¼ teaspoon white pepper
    Juice of ½ lemon (about 2 tablespoons)
  ¼ teaspoon grated lemon peel
  ½ cup crushed crackers
    Paprika

Preheat the oven to 400F (205C). Rinse and drain the fish on paper towels.

Whisk together the liquid milk, dry milk, flour, thyme, salt, and pepper in a medium saucepan until smooth. Cook over medium heat, whisking constantly, until the sauce is bubbling and thick. Stir in the lemon juice and cook, whisking constantly, 2 more minutes. Whisk in the lemon peel.

Spread ⅓ of the sauce in a gratin pan that will hold the fish in one layer. Arrange the fish in the pan, and top with the remaining sauce. Sprinkle with cracker crumbs and paprika. Bake on the top rack, until the fish flakes at the center when tested with a fork, about 18 minutes.

Makes 4 servings.

Scrod with Scalloped Tomatoes

The baked tomato "sauce" on top makes this scrod dish especially moist and flavorful. This recipe can be tripled for a buffet dish; a big stainless steel lasagna pan is just the right size.

1 tablespoon olive oil
1½ pounds scrod (in one piece), about 1-inch thick
¼ cup chopped shallots
2 medium, ripe tomatoes, sliced
2 teaspoons chopped fresh oregano or ½ teaspoon dried
  Salt and freshly ground black pepper
2 tablespoons freshly grated Parmesan cheese
1 cup fresh or ½ cup dry bread crumbs

Preheat the oven to 400F (205C).

Put the oil in a baking pan and turn the scrod over in it to coat both sides. Scatter the shallots underneath and over the scrod. Arrange the tomatoes in overlapping slices on top. Sprinkle the tomatoes with the oregano and season with salt and pepper. Top with the cheese and crumbs.

Bake on the top rack until the fish flakes at the center when tested with a fork, 20 to 25 minutes. If the crumbs become brown before the fish is cooked through, cover the dish loosely with foil.

Makes 4 servings.

Baked Haddock with Potatoes, Tomatoes, and Olives

A side dish or salad of green beans could complete the meal.

   6 plum tomatoes, sliced
   ½ cup kalamata olives, pitted and halved
   2 garlic cloves, chopped
   1 sprig of thyme, stem removed, chopped
   2 to 3 leaves fresh sage, chopped
      Salt and freshly ground pepper
   1 tablespoon olive oil
   4 potatoes, peeled and thinly sliced
1½ pounds haddock

Combine the tomatoes, olives, garlic, and herbs in a bowl. Season with salt and pepper to taste, and stir in the oil. Allow the mixture to marinate 30 minutes at room temperature.

Preheat the oven to 400F (205C). Parboil the potatoes in boiling salted water until just tender, about 5 minutes. Drain well.

Rinse and pat dry the haddock. Arrange the potatoes in overlapping slices in the bottom of an oiled baking dish that will fit the fish with 1 inch to spare all around. Lay the haddock on top. Spoon the tomato mixture over all. Bake on the middle shelf until the fish just begins to flake, 18 to 20 minutes.

Makes 4 servings.

Sea Scallop and Tomato Brochettes

Choose sea scallops (rather than the smaller bay scallops) because they are large enough to skewer.

12 ounces sea scallops
 1 garlic clove, minced (see Note, below)
 2 tablespoons olive oil
 4 strips of lemon peel, twisted to release the oil
 1 tablespoon chopped fresh marjoram or ½ teaspoon dried oregano
⅛ teaspoon salt
    Freshly ground black pepper
 8 cherry tomatoes
 2 green bell peppers, seeded and cut into large triangles
 2 cups hot cooked brown or white rice
    Lemon wedges

Rinse and drain the scallops. Combine the scallops, garlic, olive oil, lemon peel, marjoram, salt, and pepper, and allow the mixture to marinate 1 hour in the refrigerator, stirring once or twice.

Light a grill or preheat a broiler. Arrange scallops, tomatoes, and bell pepper triangles alternately on 4 metal skewers, beginning and ending with bell peppers. Double up on scallops, since there are more of them. Brush the vegetables with any remaining marinade. Broil or grill the brochettes until the pepper tips are slightly charred and the scallops are cooked through (opaque), 3 to 4 minutes per side, turning them once.

To serve, slip the scallops and vegetables off the brochettes onto a bed of rice. Serve with lemon wedges.

Makes 2 servings.

NOTE
For a less pronounced garlic flavor, don't mince it. Instead, cut the clove in half, then discard later.

Scallops with Sautéed Watercress

Peppery watercress adds zing plus the health benefits of a cruciferous vegetable to this easy entree for two. If you double the recipe, use two skillets. Scallops need lots of room if they are to brown rather than steam.

¾ pound sea scallops
2 tablespoons seasoned dry bread crumbs
2 tablespoons all-purpose flour
2 tablespoons olive oil
1 bunch of watercress, tough stems removed, chopped
Cayenne pepper (optional)
Lemon wedges

Rinse and drain the scallops. Combine the bread crumbs and flour in a plastic bag, add the scallops, and shake to coat. Shake off excess coating. Arrange the scallops on a plate and chill until ready to cook. They can be cooked immediately, but chilling sets the coating better.

Heat the oil in a 12-inch skillet over medium-high heat and sauté the scallops until they are lightly browned on both sides and cooked through, about 5 minutes. Add the watercress to the skillet and stir-fry 1 minute. Season with cayenne to taste, if desired. Serve with lemon wedges.

Makes 2 servings.

Broiled Scallops with Salsa Verde

Anchovies are high in sodium, it's true, but they're also rich in the omega-3 fatty acids. Try rinsing them in wine vinegar to make them less salty.

    Salsa Verde (see below)
¼ cup seasoned bread crumbs
¼ cup all-purpose flour
¼ cup cornmeal
1½ pounds sea scallops

Salsa Verde
1 garlic clove, peeled
2 cups well-packed flat-leaf parsley leaves (2 bunches), washed and thoroughly dried
6 anchovy fillets
1 tablespoon drained capers
¼ teaspoon freshly ground black pepper
1 tablespoon red wine vinegar
    About ½ cup olive oil

Make the Salsa Verde: With the motor running, drop the garlic down the feed tube of a food processor to mince it. Turn off the motor and remove the cover. Add the parsley, anchovies, capers, and pepper. Process until very finely chopped. With the motor running, add the vinegar, then slowly pour the oil down the feed tube until a sauce is formed, neither too thick to drop off a spoon nor runny. Stop the motor occasionally to stir and check. Makes about 1 cup.

Preheat the broiler. Mix the crumbs, flour, and cornmeal in a plastic bag. Rinse and drain the scallops. If any scallops are extra large, cut them in half. Add scallops to the bag, and shake to coat. Shake off excess coating. Lay the scallops in a single layer in an oiled shallow pan and broil them until lightly browned on one side, about 3 minutes. Turn and broil until cooked through, 2 to 3 more minutes. Serve with the sauce.

Makes 4 servings.

Scallops with Mushrooms and Brown Rice

Combining these foods makes a dish rich in brain-building B vitamins.

 3 tablespoons olive oil
 8 to 10 ounces mushrooms, cleaned and sliced
 1 shallot, chopped
 2 teaspoons chopped fresh tarragon or ½ teaspoon dried
 ⅛ teaspoon salt
    Freshly ground black pepper
 2 cups cooked brown rice
12 ounces bay scallops
 1 garlic clove, minced
 2 tablespoons chopped fresh flat-leaf parsley
    Cayenne pepper

Heat 2 tablespoons of the oil in a large skillet over high heat and sauté the mushrooms, stirring often, until their juices evaporate and they begin to brown. Add the shallot and cook 1 minute. Season the mushrooms with tarragon, salt, and black pepper. Reduce heat to medium, add the brown rice, and stir-fry 1 to 2 minutes to combine flavors. Remove the rice to a serving dish and keep it warm.

Rinse and drain the scallops. Wipe out the skillet, and add the remaining 1 tablespoon of oil. Sauté the scallops with the garlic over medium-high heat until the scallops are cooked through, about 3 minutes. Season the scallops with parsley and cayenne to taste.

To serve, make a slight well in the center of the rice and spoon the scallop mixture into it.

Makes 2 servings.

Stir-Fried Scallops with Asparagus

This Asian-inspired stir-fry is an attractive combination of colors and flavors.

1 pound sea scallops
2 tablespoons peanut oil
1 bunch scallions, cut diagonally into 2-inch pieces
4 ounces brown mushrooms, cleaned and sliced
1 pound fresh thin-stalked asparagus, cut diagonally into 2-inch pieces
4 large radishes, thinly sliced
1 slice fresh ginger, minced
2 tablespoons naturally brewed soy sauce
1 tablespoon rice vinegar

Rinse and drain the scallops. Cut any extra-large ones in half and set scallops aside.

Heat the peanut oil in a large wok or skillet over medium-high heat, and stir-fry the scallions and mushrooms until they are lightly colored. Remove them with a slotted spoon; reserve.

Stir-fry the asparagus, radishes, and ginger until the asparagus is crisp-tender, 3 to 4 minutes. Remove the vegetables with a slotted spoon; reserve.

Add more oil, if necessary. Stir-fry the scallops until they are opaque, 3 to 5 minutes. Return the other ingredients to the wok and toss with the soy sauce and vinegar. Serve immediately.

Makes 4 servings.

Spanish-Style Scallops with White Beans

A salad with tender young spinach or watercress would go nicely alongside this dish, a bonanza of B vitamins.

1½ pounds sea scallops
¾ cup seasoned dry bread crumbs
 2 tablespoons olive oil
½ cup dry white wine
 1 cup Spanish Tomato Sauce with Olives (page 322), or tomato sauce from a jar
½ teaspoon dried thyme leaves
¼ teaspoon Spicy Mixed Pepper (page 335) or black pepper
 2 cups cooked white beans (page 328) or 1 (14- to 16-oz.) can, rinsed and drained
 2 tablespoons chopped fresh flat-leaf parsley

Rinse the scallops. Cut any extra-large ones in half. Put the crumbs in a plastic bag, add the scallops, and shake the bag to coat them. Shake off any excess.

Heat the oil in a 12-inch nonstick skillet over medium-high heat, and fry the scallops until they are golden on both sides, 5 to 6 minutes. They should be opaque at the centers. Remove the scallops; reserve.

Combine the wine, tomato sauce, thyme, and pepper mix in the skillet. Bring the mixture to a boil, scraping the bottom of the skillet to loosen any brown bits. Reduce the heat and simmer 5 minutes. Add the beans and cook 5 minutes more. Return the scallops to the skillet and heat them through. Sprinkle with parsley.

Makes 4 servings.

Sautéed Lobster with Chick-pea Caponata

A richly flavored combination that's reminiscent of summer evenings by the seashore. Just add a loaf of crusty Italian bread and a bottle of light red wine.

1 large eggplant, about 1¼ pounds
1 pound cooked, shelled lobster meat
  Juice of 1 lemon
1 garlic clove, peeled and sliced
1 dried hot red chile
4 tablespoons olive oil
1 small red bell pepper, diced
2 garlic cloves, chopped
2 cups peeled, seeded, chopped fresh tomatoes, or drained canned tomatoes, chopped
1 teaspoon dried oregano
¾ teaspoon salt
¼ teaspoon freshly ground black pepper
1 (15- to 16-oz.) can chick-peas, drained and rinsed, or 2 cups cooked (page 328)
2 tablespoons red wine vinegar
1 teaspoon sugar
6 fresh basil leaves, chopped
1 tablespoon minced fresh flat-leaf parsley
  Lemon wedges, for garnish

Peel and slice the eggplant. Salt the slices and allow them to drain in a colander about 30 minutes. Rinse and press the eggplant slices to squeeze out moisture. Pat them dry between layers of paper towels. Dice the eggplant.

Cut the lobster into bite-size pieces, sprinkle with the lemon juice, and refrigerate until needed. Warm the sliced garlic and chile with 1 tablespoon of the oil in a 10-inch skillet over low heat, 5 minutes. Do not brown the garlic. Let stand while cooking the eggplant.

Heat 2 tablespoons of the oil in a separate 12-inch skillet over medium-high heat and stir-fry the eggplant until it begins to brown. Add the 1 remaining tablespoon of oil, bell pepper, and chopped garlic. Sauté over low heat, stirring often, 3 minutes. Don't let the garlic brown. Add the tomatoes, oregano, salt, and pepper to the eggplant, and cook over low heat, stirring occasionally, until the mixture is quite thick, about 20 to 25 minutes. Add the chick-peas, vinegar, sugar, and basil, and cook 5 to 10 minutes, until the eggplant is tender. Stir in the parsley. Let this mixture cool until it's just warm or room temperature.

Warm the lobster meat in the 10-inch skillet with the sliced garlic and hot chile. Discard the garlic and chile.

To serve, spoon a helping of caponata on each of 4 plates. Arrange the lobster on the side, dividing it equally among the plates. Garnish with lemon wedges.

Makes 4 servings, with some leftover caponata.

Shrimp with Chiles and Lime

This shrimp combination includes lots of phytochemicals that build a stronger immune system.

2 tablespoons olive oil
2 large green onions (the size of plums) or 1 bunch scallions, chopped
2 mild green chiles, seeded and cut into chunks
1 red bell pepper, seeded and cut into chunks
1 pound large raw shrimp, shelled and deveined, or frozen cooked shrimp, thawed
   Freshly ground black pepper
   Juice of 1 lime
   Lime wedges, for garnish

Heat the oil in a 12-inch skillet over medium-high heat and sauté the onions, chiles, and bell pepper until they are crisp-tender, 3 to 5 minutes. Add the raw shrimp and sauté until they all turn pink, about 5 minutes, or add thawed cooked shrimp and sauté 2 minutes to combine flavors. Season with black pepper and sprinkle with lime juice. Serve at once with a garnish of lime wedges.

Makes 4 servings.

Greek-Style Shrimp with Tomatoes and Feta

Brown basmati rice makes a nice accompaniment to this
Mediterranean entree.

1 pound extra-large raw shrimp (about 40)
2 tablespoons olive oil
1 small red onion, finely chopped
1 celery stalk, finely diced
2 cups peeled, seeded, chopped fresh tomatoes
1 teaspoon chopped fresh thyme or ¼ teaspoon dried
¼ teaspoon salt
⅛ teaspoon freshly ground pepper
1 cup (about 4 ounces) crumbled feta cheese

Peel the shrimp and remove the black vein along the back. Rinse and pat dry the shrimp.

Heat the oil in a large skillet over medium heat and sauté the onion and celery until they are translucent, about 5 minutes. Add the tomatoes, thyme, salt, and pepper. Simmer, uncovered, until thickened to a light sauce consistency, 5 to 10 minutes.

Add the shrimp, cover, and simmer until the shrimp curl up and turn pink, 3 to 5 minutes. Stir in the feta cheese and remove from the heat.

Makes 4 servings.

Scampi and Zucchini

Deliciously simple. Buy cooked, cleaned shrimp at a reliable fish store, and you can have this entree on the table in 10 minutes. Or if you prefer, cook and clean the raw shrimp ahead of time (page 336).

2 tablespoons olive oil
1 red bell pepper, seeded and cut into 2-inch strips
2 small zucchini, cut into ¼-inch half-rounds
1 to 2 garlic cloves, minced
1 pound cooked, shelled, deveined shrimp (page 336)
   Juice of 1 lemon, about ¼ cup
1 tablespoon minced fresh flat-leaf parsley
   Freshly ground black pepper

Heat the olive oil in a large wok or skillet over medium-high heat, and stir-fry the bell pepper and zucchini until they are crisp-tender, 3 to 5 minutes. Add the garlic and shrimp and cook 1 minute more. Season with lemon juice, parsley, and pepper.

Makes 4 servings.

Poultry Dishes—Easy Protein for Maximum Energy

Protein, from the Greek word *proteios*, means "of prime importance"—and so it is, essential to every part and process of the body, so abundantly present that it is second only to water. Ten to 12 percent of one's daily calories should come from protein.

In this country of major meat eaters, it's surprising to learn that many people over the age of fifty-five are not getting their healthy share of protein, just when they need it most. Older adults need protein for at least three important reasons: to maximize their energy, to support their immune systems, and to maintain the body's water balance. If protein levels fall too low, edema, (fluid retention) can result. Those who have adopted a vegetarian lifestyle will have to manage menu planning carefully to get all the complete protein required, but the rest of the population has easy access to a plentiful supply in poultry.

One of the reasons older adults may veer away from meat is the fear of fat and cholesterol. But moderation, not abstinence, may be the best answer. When poultry is baked, braised, or poached and served without its skin in moderate portions, you won't have to worry about clogging your arteries. Half a chicken breast, skinned and poached, contains 3 grams of fat, of which only 1 gram is saturated, and 65 milligrams of cholesterol. Compare this to 3 ounces of well-done lean hamburger, which contains 14 grams of fat, of which 5 are saturated, and 84 milligrams of cholesterol. The more you substitute white meat for red, the healthier your heart will be. And that's not all. In a wide study of registered nurses published in the *New England Journal of Medicine,* women who substituted lean chicken and fish for beef, pork, and lamb were 50 percent less likely to develop colon cancer.

Not all poultry products, however, are low fat. A word of caution is needed about ground turkey: It's not automatically less fatty. Some ground turkey has just as much fat as ground beef. You need to check the percentage of fat in the ground meat you buy. Look for lean or extra-lean ground turkey, and you'll be enjoying a real low-fat alternative to the heart-stopping big beef burger that's so popular in America.

And a second caution about handling. A virtual epidemic of salmonella has invaded the poultry industry in recent years, probably due to the unhealthy crowded conditions in which the birds are raised. Some simple commonsense measures will keep you safe from this scourge. Wash raw poultry in cold salted water before cooking (I like to use kosher salt), rinse in fresh water, and pat dry with paper towels. Use hot soapy water to wash your hands and all surfaces that come in contact with raw poultry. Thaw poultry in the refrigerator, not on the drain board. In a chicken-thawing emergency, use the microwave. Cook poultry until it's no longer pink. And last, refrigerate leftover poultry promptly, especially that big bird you have at Thanksgiving. Follow these few rules and relax! Poultry is a super dish, and not just for its protein.

Chicken and turkey are great sources of B vitamins as well as protein, including that vital B_{12}, which protects the nervous system and mental capacity as we age, and which can be found only in animal foods. In addition, poultry offers zinc for immunity and wound healing, selenium for cancer prevention, and potassium for the heart.

From the cook's point of view, few foods are as versatile as chicken—and turkey, too, now that supermarkets are selling it in convenient cuts. The way chicken or turkey can be teamed up with other superfoods, like vegetables and grains, makes them a boon to healthy meal planning.

Herbed Chicken and Roasted Vegetable Casserole

An easy-to-prepare dinner for six that cooks in a little less than an hour with only one stir. Relax and put your feet up!

  2 large shallots, sliced
  2 green bell peppers, seeded and cut into strips
  2 carrots, cut diagonally into 1-inch-thick slices
1½ pounds (3 large) red potatoes, unpeeled and cut lengthwise into quarters
  6 chicken thighs or leg quarters, skinned
  ½ cup tomato juice
  2 tablespoons chopped fresh herbs: basil, rosemary, sage, and/or thyme leaves
     Salt and freshly ground pepper
  2 tablespoons olive oil
  1 medium zucchini, cut crosswise into 8 rounds

Preheat the oven to 375F (190C).

Lightly oil a large oven-to-table gratin or flat casserole dish (13 × 9-inch). Layer the vegetables (except zucchini) in the following order: shallots, bell peppers, carrots, and potatoes. Arrange the chicken on top. Pour the tomato juice over all. Sprinkle with the fresh herbs and salt and pepper to taste. Drizzle with the oil.

Bake, uncovered, 30 minutes. Add the zucchini and stir. Bake until the vegetables are tender and the chicken cooked through, 20 to 30 minutes more.

Makes 6 servings.

Chicken Divan-in-a-Pan

A light, no-fuss version of the classic baked chicken-and-broccoli dish. Oven-Baked Brown and Wild Rice Pilaf (page 141) and a sliced tomato salad would round out an attractive, balanced menu.

　8　stalks fresh broccoli or 1 package (10-oz.) frozen broccoli
1¼ to 1½ pounds boneless, skinless chicken breasts
　¼　cup all-purpose flour
　2　tablespoons olive oil
　5　ounces mushrooms, cleaned and sliced
　1　shallot, chopped
　1　celery stalk, diced small
　1　cup Chicken-Mushroom Stock (page 333) or canned broth
　¼　teaspoon salt
　⅛　teaspoon white pepper
　1　teaspoon chopped fresh thyme or ¼ teaspoon dried
　3　tablespoons nonfat dry milk
1½　tablespoons instant flour, such as Wondra
　½　cup milk

Cook the broccoli in a 12-inch nonstick skillet. For fresh broccoli, add about 1 inch of water and a few dashes of salt. Bring to a boil, cover, and simmer until the broccoli is crisp-tender, about 5 minutes. For frozen broccoli, follow package directions. Remove and reserve the broccoli.

Cut the chicken breasts crosswise into ½-inch-wide slices. Put them in a plastic bag with the all-purpose flour and shake to coat the chicken. Shake off excess flour.

Rinse and dry the skillet. Heat 1 tablespoon of oil in the skillet over medium heat and sauté the mushrooms, shallot, and celery, stirring often, until lightly browned, 5 to 8 minutes. Remove the vegetables; reserve.

Add the remaining 1 tablespoon of oil to the skillet and brown the chicken on both sides over medium-high heat. (If your skillet is smaller than 12 inches, you will have to do this in batches.) Add the stock, salt, pepper, and thyme, scraping the bottom of the pan to loosen any brown bits. Add the cooked celery mixture, cover, and simmer until the chicken is cooked through, 10 to 15 minutes.

Stir the dry milk and instant flour into the liquid milk, and pour it into the pan. Cook, stirring constantly but gently, until the pan juices are thickened and smooth. Return the broccoli to the pan and heat through.

Makes 4 servings.

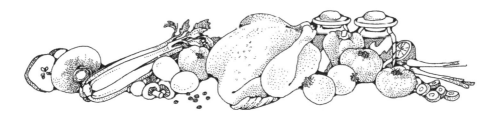

Chili Chicken with Corn and Pinto Beans

Even if you're not going the vegetarian route, it makes sense to "stretch" smaller meat portions with great vegetables. Corn and pinto beans in this dish are both high-fiber foods, and there's lots of vitamin C, too, in the peppers, chile, and tomatoes.

1 pound boneless, skinless chicken breasts, cut into 1-inch chunks
½ cup all-purpose flour
  About 2 tablespoons olive oil
1 large yellow onion, chopped
1 large mild green chile, seeded and diced
1 red bell pepper, seeded and diced
1 garlic clove, minced
2 cups Chicken-Mushroom Stock (page 333) or canned broth
1 (14- to 16-oz.) can ground tomatoes (not puree)
2 teaspoons minced fresh oregano or ½ teaspoon dried
2 teaspoons chili powder
1 teaspoon ground cumin
  Pinch of ground cinnamon
½ teaspoon salt
¼ teaspoon freshly ground black pepper
1½ cups fresh or frozen corn kernels
1 (14- to 16-oz.) can pinto or shell beans, drained and rinsed, or 2 cups cooked (page 328)
¼ cup chopped fresh cilantro or flat-leaf parsley

Put the chicken into a plastic bag with the flour. Hold the bag closed, and shake it to coat the chicken. Shake off excess flour.

Heat the oil in a Dutch oven or large heavy pot and brown the chicken pieces, stirring often. Remove them with a slotted spoon; reserve. Adding more oil to the pot, if necessary, sauté the onion, chile, and bell pepper 5 minutes, until softened. Add the garlic during the last minute.

Add the stock, tomatoes, oregano, chili powder, cumin, cinnamon, salt, and black pepper. Cover and simmer, stirring often, until the chicken is cooked through, 15 to 20 minutes.

Add the corn and beans. Return to a simmer, and cook 5 minutes longer. Stir in the cilantro or parsley.

Makes 4 servings.

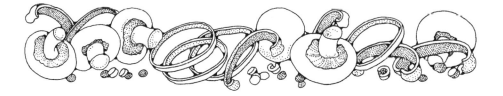

Dijon Chicken with Roasted Cabbage

This is another way to serve cruciferous cabbage. The vegetable takes on a different and pleasing flavor when roasted with chicken.

⅓ cup nonfat plain yogurt
1 tablespoon Dijon mustard
2 cups fresh bread crumbs from 2 slices crustless Italian bread
4 large chicken thighs, skinned
2 teaspoons chopped fresh rosemary or ½ teaspoon dried
8 small wedges cabbage (½ of a large head)
   Olive oil
   Salt and freshly ground black pepper

Preheat the oven to 375F (190C). Oil a large gratin or baking pan.

Mix together the yogurt and mustard. Put the bread crumbs on a sheet of waxed paper. Coat each of the thighs with some of the mustard mixture, then dip into the bread crumbs to coat completely on both sides. This messy job is best done with the hands in order to get an even, complete coating.

Arrange the chicken in the center of the oiled pan, allowing room for the cabbage. Sprinkle with rosemary. Arrange the cabbage wedges around the chicken. Drizzle a little olive oil over each cabbage wedge and salt and pepper them to taste. Bake on the middle rack until the chicken is golden brown and cooked through, about 45 minutes. Do not turn the chicken, but loosen the cabbage from the bottom of the pan with a fork about halfway through the cooking time.

Makes 4 servings.

Chicken and Vegetables with Japanese Noodles

This stir-fry, ready in minutes, is a meal in itself—a good choice for easy after-work cooking.

> About 3 tablespoons peanut or canola oil
> 2 cups chopped bok choy
> 1 bunch scallions, cut diagonally into ½-inch pieces
> 1 red bell pepper, seeded and cut into small triangles
> 1 small zucchini, quartered lengthwise and cut into 1-inch-thick chunks
> 1 garlic clove, minced
> 1 pound boneless, skinless, chicken breast, cut into ½-inch strips
> 2 tablespoons cornstarch
> 1 cup chicken broth
> 2 tablespoons regular or low-sodium naturally brewed soy sauce, or to taste
> 1 tablespoon rice vinegar
> 1 teaspoon sugar
> 8 ounces Japanese noodles or thin linguine

Heat 1 tablespoon of the oil in a large wok or skillet over medium-high heat, and stir-fry the bok choy and scallions until crisp-tender, about 2 minutes. Remove the vegetables with a slotted spoon; reserve. Add 1 teaspoon of the oil to wok, if needed. Add the bell pepper and zucchini and stir-fry until crisp-tender, about 3 minutes. Add the garlic during the last minute. Remove the vegetables; reserve.

Toss the chicken pieces with the cornstarch. Add 2 teaspoons more oil to the wok, if needed, and stir fry the chicken until cooked through, 4 to 7 minutes. Mix the broth with the soy sauce, vinegar, and sugar. Add to the wok and bring to a boil, stirring until bubbling and slightly thickened (from the cornstarch on the chicken). Return the vegetables to the wok and heat through. Taste and correct seasoning, adding more soy sauce, if desired.

Meanwhile, cook the noodles according to package directions and drain. In a large serving dish, toss the noodles with the chicken and vegetables.

Makes 4 servings.

Chicken and Vegetable Ragout

An easy supper dish with a French influence.

    2 tablespoons olive oil
    1 yellow bell pepper, seeded and diced
    1 green bell pepper, seeded and diced
    ¼ cup chopped shallots
1½ pounds boneless, skinless chicken breasts, cut crosswise into ½-
      inch-thick slices
    1 large (about ¾-pound) zucchini, quartered lengthwise and cut into
      1-inch-thick chunks
    2 medium carrots, cut diagonally into ½-inch-thick slices
1½ cups French Tomato Sauce (page 323) or tomato sauce from a jar
    ½ cup chicken broth
    1 teaspoon *herbes de Provence* (available in specialty stores) or ¼
      teaspoon each of the following dried herbs: fennel, rosemary,
      thyme, tarragon, and basil
    ¼ teaspoon salt
    ⅛ teaspoon freshly ground black pepper
    8 slices French baguette
      Additional olive oil, for brushing bread
    1 garlic clove, halved

Heat the oil in a large skillet over medium heat and stir-fry the peppers and shallots until sizzling and fragrant, about 3 minutes. Add the chicken and stir-fry until the meat is no longer pink, another 5 minutes. Add the zucchini, carrots, tomato sauce, broth, *herbes de Provence*, salt, and black pepper. Cook with lid slightly ajar, stirring occasionally, until the vegetables are tender and the chicken is cooked through, 8 to 10 minutes. Taste and correct seasoning, adding more salt or pepper, if desired.

Brush the baguette slices with olive oil and rub them with the garlic clove. Toast them under a broiler, watching closely to prevent burning. Serve the ragout in bowls with the toasted bread.

Makes 4 servings.

All-American Crusty, Not Fatty, Fried Chicken with Garlic, Oregano, and Lime

Using a minimum of oil, as this recipe does, requires very slow and patient frying to yield a crispy crust, about 15 minutes per side. Sweet Potato and Apple Casserole makes a lovely side dish (page 226).

4 to 6 large chicken thighs, skinned
   All-purpose flour, for coating
2 tablespoons olive oil
   Salt and freshly ground black pepper
   Dried oregano
2 garlic cloves, chopped
   Juice of 1 to 2 limes
   Lime wedges

Coat the chicken with flour, shaking off excess.

Heat the oil in a 10-inch nonstick skillet for 4 thighs or a 12-inch one for 6 thighs over medium-low heat. Fry the chicken on one side, with lid ajar, until it is golden brown, about 15 minutes. Salt and pepper it to taste. Turn chicken, sprinkle it liberally with the oregano and chopped garlic. Again, with lid ajar, slowly fry the chicken until the pieces are nicely crisp and the meat is just cooked to the bone, not pink but still juicy, about 15 minutes more.

Remove the chicken to warm dinner plates, sprinkle with lime juice, and serve immediately. Pass more lime wedges on the side.

Makes 4 to 6 servings.

Chicken Florentine with Walnuts

Walnuts are one of the few nonfish sources of those heart-healthy omega-3 fatty acids.

1 (1-lb. bag) fresh spinach
4 boneless, skinless chicken breast halves
   All-purpose flour, for coating
   About 2 tablespoons olive oil
1 teaspoon chopped fresh oregano or ¼ teaspoon dried
   Salt and freshly ground pepper
1 bunch scallions, cut diagonally into 1-inch lengths
1 cup Chicken-Mushroom Stock (page 333) or canned broth
2 tablespoons fresh lemon juice
1 tablespoon cornstarch
⅛ teaspoon white pepper
½ cup walnut halves or pieces
   Lemon wedges, for garnish

Wash the spinach well, remove tough stems, and chop it coarsely. Steam spinach in just the water that clings to the leaves in a covered 12-inch skillet over medium heat, until wilted, about 5 minutes. Remove the spinach with a slotted spoon. Clean and dry the skillet.

With a wooden mallet or the flat side of a chef's knife, pound the chicken pieces to flatten them slightly. Coat them with the flour, shaking off excess. Heat 2 tablespoons oil in the skillet over medium heat and fry the chicken until golden. Turn chicken and sprinkle with oregano, and salt and pepper to taste. Fry until cooked through, about 7 minutes total cooking time. Remove the chicken and keep it warm.

Add the scallions and a little more oil, if needed, to the skillet and sauté them until limp and tender, 3 minutes. Mix the stock, lemon juice, and cornstarch until smooth, and pour the mixture into the skillet. Cook over medium-high heat, scraping up the browned bits and stirring constantly, until the sauce is bubbling and thickened. Season with white pepper. Stir in the walnuts and simmer 3 minutes.

To serve, reheat the spinach. Divide the spinach among 4 plates, top with chicken, and pour ¼ of the sauce and walnuts over each serving. Garnish with lemon wedges.

Makes 4 servings.

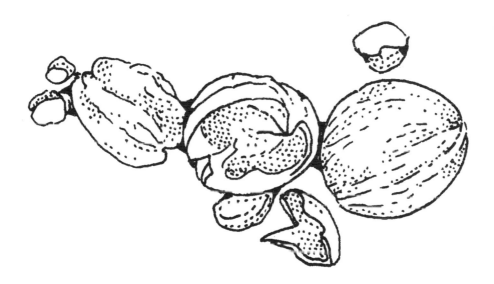

Confetti Chicken

This dish is a "natural" for a buffet dinner. If you double the recipe, use two skillets; the chicken needs space to brown properly. Hot cooked brown basmati rice is a good accompaniment.

1½ pounds boneless, skinless chicken breasts, cut into 1-inch cubes
⅓ cup all-purpose flour
½ teaspoon ground cumin
½ teaspoon ground coriander
¼ teaspoon salt
⅛ teaspoon freshly ground black pepper
 About 2 tablespoons olive oil
1 green bell pepper, seeded and diced small
1 red bell pepper, seeded and diced small
1 jalapeño chile, seeded and minced (see Note below)
2 large shallots, minced
1 tablespoon minced fresh flat-leaf parsley
⅓ cup canned juice-packed pineapple tidbits, drained

Put the chicken into a plastic bag with the flour, cumin, coriander, salt, and black pepper. Hold the bag closed, and shake it to coat the chicken. Shake off excess flour.

Heat the oil in a 12-inch skillet over medium heat, and brown the chicken in two batches until lightly golden on both sides, about 5 minutes per batch. Remove first batch with slotted spoon and reserve while cooking second batch.

Return first batch of chicken to chicken in skillet. Add the bell peppers, chile, shallots, and more oil, if needed, to chicken. Sauté, stirring occasionally, until the chicken is cooked through and the peppers are crisp-tender, about 10 minutes. Stir in the parsley and pineapple; heat through. Taste a piece of chicken; add more salt and pepper, if desired.

Makes 4 servings.

NOTE

Wear rubber gloves to protect your hands from the oil when seeding and chopping hot chiles. To prevent irritation, never rub your eyes with your fingers after handling hot chiles.

Braised Chicken Breasts with Peppers and Fennel

Virginia's Wild Rice with Mushrooms, Onion, and Cream makes a perfect accompaniment (page 148).

4 boneless, skinless chicken breast halves
   All-purpose flour, for coating
2 tablespoons olive oil
1 large shallot, minced
1 yellow bell pepper, seeded and diced
1 red bell pepper, seeded and diced
1 cup chopped fennel or celery
   Salt and freshly ground black pepper
¼ teaspoon dried thyme
¼ teaspoon dried rosemary or marjoram

Coat the chicken in flour, shaking off excess. Heat the oil in a 12-inch skillet over medium heat and sauté chicken until lightly browned on one side. Scatter the shallot, bell peppers, and fennel around the chicken. If they don't fit at first, they will as they soften. Add salt and pepper to taste and sprinkle the chicken with thyme and rosemary. Cover, leaving lid slightly ajar. Slowly braise over low heat until chicken is cooked through and the vegetables are crisp-tender, stirring vegetables once or twice, 20 to 25 minutes total cooking time.

Makes 4 servings.

Mediterranean Chicken Pie

An all-in-one dinner for a hungry family or a substantial buffet dish, this pie uses skinless, boneless chicken tenders. These are chicken tenderloins, yet they cost less than boned breasts. Some markets will trim off the short piece of attached gristle; if not, it's easy to do with a sharp knife.

If you don't want to make your own pizza dough, you can buy ready-made dough in many supermarkets.

   Pizza Dough (page 184)
 1 tablespoon olive oil
 1 small yellow onion, chopped
 1 pound chicken tenders, gristle removed, then cut into 1-inch pieces
 1 green or red bell pepper, seeded and cut into 1-inch pieces
 4 to 5 ounces mushrooms, cleaned and sliced (optional)
 1 clove garlic, minced
 1 (16-oz.) can Italian plum tomatoes, chopped, with juice
 1 pound russet potatoes, cut into 1-inch pieces
 1 medium carrot, cut crosswise into ½-inch-thick slices
 ½ teaspoon dried Italian herbs, or pinches of dried rosemary, oregano, basil, and thyme
 ½ teaspoon salt
 ⅛ teaspoon freshly ground black pepper
 3 tablespoons instant flour, such as Wondra
 1 cup Chicken-Mushroom Stock (page 333) or canned broth
 1 cup fresh shelled or frozen green peas

Make the pizza dough through its first rising. Punch it down and roll it out ¼ inch thick. With a floured biscuit cutter, cut the dough into rounds. Let the rounds rise while making the pot-pie filling.

Preheat the oven to 400F (205C). Heat the oil in a Dutch oven or 12-inch skillet over medium heat and fry the onion 1 minute. Add the chicken and stir-fry until it's partly browned. Add the bell pepper and mushrooms, if using, and fry over medium-high heat, stirring often, until lightly colored, 3 minutes. Reduce the heat and add the garlic; cook 1 minute. Add the tomatoes, potatoes, carrot, herbs, salt, and pepper. Simmer, covered, until the chicken is cooked through and the vegetables are tender, about 10 minutes.

Mix the flour into the cold stock until blended. Stir flour mixture into the pan, and cook over medium heat, stirring constantly, until the sauce bubbles and thickens. Stir in the peas and cook 3 minutes.

Spoon the mixture into a 13 × 9-inch gratin pan or nonreactive baking dish. The liquid level should be below the chicken and vegetables. Place the dough rounds on top. Bake until the rounds are golden and the stew is bubbling throughout, about 30 minutes.

Makes about 6 servings.

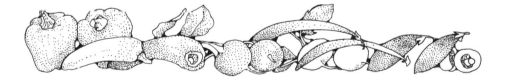

Chicken Tagine

A tagine is a North African stew. The rich flavors of cinnamon and prunes, plus antioxidants and fiber in sweet potatoes and chick-peas, make this oven-baked casserole a truly super dish.

1   tablespoon olive oil
4   large skinless chicken thighs
1   large yellow onion, chopped
1   (16-oz.) can plum tomatoes, chopped, with juice
1   (14- to 16-oz.) can chick-peas, drained and rinsed, or 2 cups cooked (page 328)
1   pound sweet potatoes, cut into chunks
½   cup fresh orange juice
4   strips orange peel (with no white pith)
1   cinnamon stick
1   dried hot red chile
1   teaspoon ground cumin
½   teaspoon salt
¼   teaspoon freshly ground black pepper
½   cup pitted prunes

Preheat the oven to 350F (175C).

Heat the oil over medium heat in a Dutch oven or other rangetop-to-oven pan and brown the chicken on both sides, in batches if necessary. Add the onion and cook 3 minutes.

Add the tomatoes, chick-peas, sweet potatoes, orange juice, orange peel, cinnamon, chile, cumin, salt, and pepper. Bring to a simmer, stirring to loosen any brown bits on the bottom of the pan. Cover and bake on the middle rack of the oven about 45 minutes, stirring once or twice and checking liquid. Add the prunes and bake 5 to 10 minutes or until the chicken is cooked through and potatoes are tender.

Remove the cinnamon stick and chile before serving.

Makes 4 servings.

Braised Chicken with Oranges and Almonds

*Like all of nature's seed foods, almonds are a rich source of nutrients.
They contain boron, riboflavin, and copper.*

- 4   boneless, skinless chicken breast halves
    All-purpose flour, for coating
- 2   tablespoons olive oil
- ¼   cup sliced shallots
- ¼   cup whole blanched almonds
    Salt and pepper
- 4   small sprigs of fresh thyme
    About 1 cup Chicken-Mushroom Stock (page 333) or canned broth
- 2   medium-to-small navel oranges, peel and pith removed, cut into segments

Coat the chicken in flour; shake off excess. Heat the oil in a 12-inch skillet over medium heat, and brown the chicken, turning. When the second side is almost brown, scatter the shallots and almonds around the chicken pieces, and sauté (but don't brown) about 2 minutes, stirring them frequently. Salt and pepper the chicken. Put a sprig of thyme on each chicken piece. Add the stock and braise the chicken, with cover slightly ajar, until it's cooked through, about 15 minutes. If necessary, add more stock.

Add the oranges, and cook just long enough to warm them in the pan juices. Divide the chicken, oranges, and nuts among 4 dinner plates, and serve at once.

Makes 4 servings.

Braised Turkey Tenderloins with Red Bell Peppers

A turkey tenderloin is a small (about ¾-pound) tongue-shaped portion of the bird that corresponds to a whole beef tenderloin.

1 tablespoon olive oil
2 turkey tenderloins (about 1¼ pounds total)
2 red bell peppers, seeded and cut into strips
1 bunch scallions, sliced diagonally into 2-inch pieces
4 thin strips lemon peel (without any white pith)
1 cup water
½ teaspoon dried marjoram leaves
¼ teaspoon dried thyme
¼ teaspoon salt
    Freshly ground pepper
2 teaspoons cornstarch stirred into ½ cup cold water
    Cooked rice or couscous

Preheat the oven to 375F (190C).

Heat the oil in a Dutch oven or flameproof baking dish over medium heat and lightly brown the tenderloins on both sides, turning as needed. When the second side is browning, add the bell peppers and scallions. Cook until the vegetables are sizzling and fragrant. Add the lemon peel, water, herbs, salt, and pepper. Bring mixture to a simmer, cover the pan, and place on the middle rack. Bake 45 minutes or until the turkey is cooked through and tender.

Remove the turkey to a platter. Bring the liquid to a boil on the range-top. Stir in cornstarch mixture and cook, stirring constantly, until the sauce bubbles and thickens. Reduce the heat, and simmer 2 to 3 minutes, stirring occasionally.

Let the turkey stand 5 to 10 minutes. Cut turkey diagonally into about 1-inch-thick slices, surround the slices with the peppers, and pour the sauce over all. Serve with rice or couscous.

Makes 4 servings.

Turkey Meat Loaf with Dijon Topping

This basic meat loaf mix can also be used to make tiny meatballs to cook in soup or larger ones to fry as sandwich burgers with an Italian flavor.

1 slice fresh Italian bread
1 shallot, peeled and halved
4 or 5 sprigs of fresh parsley, stemmed and chopped
4 or 5 leaves of fresh basil, stemmed and chopped, or ½ teaspoon
  dried Italian herbs
2 tablespoons freshly grated Parmesan cheese
½ teaspoon salt
⅛ teaspoon freshly ground pepper
1 large egg
1¼ pounds lean ground turkey breast
½ cup plain nonfat yogurt
1 tablespoon Dijon mustard
1 teaspoon cornstarch

Preheat the oven to 350F (175C).

Processor method: Make bread crumbs by tossing pieces of bread down the feed tube with the motor running. Remove the crumbs. Combine the shallot and herbs in the work bowl and pulse to mince them. Add the bread crumbs, cheese, and seasonings; process to mix. Add the egg and ground turkey. Pulse until just blended.

By hand: Mince the shallots and herbs. Wet the bread and press out the moisture. Blend the shallot mixture and bread with the cheese, salt, pepper, egg, and ground turkey, breaking up the bread pieces until the mixture is well blended.

Spoon the mixture into a 9 × 5-inch loaf pan. Whisk together the yogurt, mustard, and cornstarch until well blended. Spread the mixture over the meat loaf. Bake on the middle rack 35 to 40 minutes or until cooked through with no pink at the center, 165 to 170F (75C) on an instant-read thermometer.

Makes 6 servings.

Turkey and Corn Bread Cobbler

Green Salad with Kiwifruit and Shaved Parmesan (page 253) makes an interesting accompaniment to this down-home main dish.

  1 tablespoon olive oil
  2 turkey tenderloins (about 1¼ pounds total)
  1 green bell pepper, seeded and cut into strips
  1 yellow onion, diced
1½ cups Chicken-Mushroom Stock (page 333), canned broth, or prepared bouillon
  2 large carrots, cut diagonally into 1-inch-thick slices
  1 teaspoon chopped fresh tarragon or ¼ teaspoon dried
  ¼ teaspoon salt
  ⅛ teaspoon freshly ground black pepper
  1 tablespoon cornstarch stirred into ½ cup cold water

Corn Bread Topping
  ½ cup cornmeal, preferably whole-grain
  ½ cup unbleached all-purpose flour
  ½ teaspoon baking powder
  ¼ teaspoon salt
  ⅛ teaspoon cayenne pepper
  ¼ cup dried cranberries (optional), plumped in hot water
  ½ cup milk
  1 egg, beaten
  1 tablespoon canola oil

Heat the oil in an ovenproof skillet or Dutch oven over medium heat, and lightly brown the tenderloins. When the second side is browning, add the bell pepper and onion. Cook until the vegetables are sizzling and fragrant. Add the stock, carrots, tarragon, salt, and pepper. Bring the mixture to a simmer. Cover and simmer until the turkey is cooked through and tender, about 30 minutes. Remove and dice the turkey. Measure the cooking liquid; if less than 1 cup, add water to make 1 cup and pour into pan.

Bring the cooking liquid and carrots to a simmer, and stir in the corn-starch mixture. Cook, stirring constantly, until sauce is bubbling and thickened. Add the diced turkey and simmer 3 minutes.

Preheat the oven to 400F (205C). Mix together the dry ingredients for the topping. Stir in the dried cranberries, if using. Mix the liquid ingredients in a separate bowl, and add them all at once to the dry ingredients. Stir until just blended. Drop the batter by tablespoons over the turkey and vegetables. Bake 25 to 30 minutes, until the topping is golden brown.

Makes 4 servings.

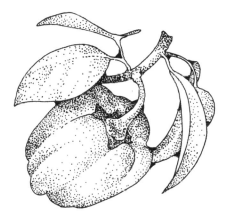

Turkey Cutlets with Balsamic Vinegar Sauce

Turkey is a surprisingly nutritious meat choice. Besides the iron and B$_{12}$ you would expect to find in meat, turkey is also a great source of zinc, chromium, and niacin.

1 large egg
1 large egg white
2 tablespoons water
¼ teaspoon salt
⅛ teaspoon freshly ground black pepper
⅓ cup unbleached all-purpose flour
1 cup seasoned dry bread crumbs
8 turkey cutlets
  About 3 tablespoons olive oil
1 garlic clove, peeled and halved
1 cup Chicken-Mushroom Stock (page 333) or canned broth
2 tablespoons balsamic vinegar

Beat together the egg, egg white, water, salt, and pepper in a shallow bowl. Arrange a sheet of waxed paper on either side of the bowl. Put the flour on one sheet, the crumbs on the other. Using 2 forks, dip the cutlets first in flour, then in the egg mixture, then in crumbs. Arrange the cutlets on a platter in one layer and chill to set the coating, about 30 minutes.

Heat about 1½ tablespoons of the oil in a 12-inch skillet over medium-high heat until shimmering hot. Add ½ of the garlic and 4 cutlets. Reduce heat to medium-low and fry the cutlets until golden on both sides. Remove them to a platter and keep warm. Remove and discard the browned garlic and add the remaining garlic to the skillet. Add more oil, heat it, and cook the remaining 4 cutlets. Remove them to the platter.

Remove and discard the remaining garlic. Add the stock and vinegar to the skillet. Cook over high heat until reduced to about ¼ cup. Pour the sauce over the cutlets and serve.

Makes 4 servings.

Turkey Chili

Chili is easily doubled, cooked ahead, and reheated, and all those won-derful qualities make a good "Superbowl watching" dish.

    2 tablespoons canola oil
    1 large onion, chopped
    1 to 2 jalapeño chiles, seeded and minced (see Note,
       page 120)
    1 garlic clove, minced
1½ pounds lean ground turkey
    2 cups peeled, seeded, chopped fresh tomatoes or 1 (14- to 16-oz.)
       can tomatoes, undrained
    1 cup Chicken-Mushroom Stock (page 333) or canned broth
    1 tablespoon chopped fresh cilantro or 1 teaspoon dried
    1 teaspoon ground cumin
    1 teaspoon dried oregano
    ½ teaspoon salt
    1 (14-oz.) can pinto beans, drained and rinsed, or 1½ cups cooked
       (page 328)
    1 (14-oz.) can chick-peas, drained and rinsed, or 1½ cups cooked
       (page 328)
    4 scallions, chopped

Heat the oil in a Dutch oven or large heavy pot over medium heat and sauté the onion and chile until they begin to color, 3 minutes. Add the garlic and sauté 1 minute more. Add the ground turkey, breaking it up with a spatula, and sauté until it's no longer pink, 5 minutes. Add the tomatoes, stock, cilantro, cumin, oregano, and salt. Bring to a simmer and cook, uncovered, 5 minutes, stirring often.

Add the beans and chick-peas, and cook, covered, stirring often, 10 minutes. Transfer to a serving dish and sprinkle with the scallions.

Makes 4 servings.

Nourishing Grains, Pastas, and Breads

❧❧

At the broad base of the Food Guide Pyramid are the nourishing grains, pastas, and breads that are an abundant source of B vitamins, carbohydrates, and fiber. The United States Department of Agriculture recommends that we consume six to eleven servings from this food group daily. Fortunately, these are among our favorite foods. Although some of us may need prompting with brussels sprouts and turnip greens, few need to be urged to eat pizza, pasta, and the ever-popular sandwich.

Not all grains, however, are created equal. In order to take advantage of all the body and brain power this food group has to offer, you need to "separate the wheat from the chaff" or, more precisely, to separate the whole wheat from the refined grains, at least some of the time. Whole grains include the outer cellulose layer (bran) and the germ, where the plant has stored most of its vitamins, minerals, and fiber. Oatmeal is perhaps the only grain in which the unrefined form is the most widely available. "Enriching" flour, rice, cereal, and bread sounds good, but it simply means that the manufacturer has compensated for some of the important B vitamins that were lost in the refining process, but not, alas, for the fiber. And we need that fiber—soluble fiber for the heart, insoluble fiber for the digestive system.

All the foods in this group, however, whether whole-grain or not, are a first-class source of complex carbohydrates. The useful "carbs" provide an energy boost that can be readily put to use not only by the body

133

but also by the brain and nervous system. Physical stamina depends on carbohydrates, but that's not all. A calm, cheerful mood can also be induced by a high-carb snack.

The notion that these "starchy" foods are more fattening than foods in other groups, notably proteins, has been called a myth by leading nutritionists. Nevertheless, it's a theme that keeps cropping up in trendy diet programs. Yet controlled studies have clearly shown that a high-carbohydrate diet not only results in weight loss, it also keeps dieters from feeling deprived, cranky, and hungry. But carbohydrates do more than give dieters the pleasant feeling of having eaten something substantial. Because the body stores them less efficiently, the process of digesting carbohydrates actually burns more calories than digesting fats.

Every ethnic cuisine has its favorites among the starchy grain foods, from cornmeal in Mexico and rice in Asia and Spain to the myriad forms of pasta in Italy and the great wheat breads of Northern Europe. Because our country is a "melting pot," we have access to the marvelous variety of these traditions. Some of the specialty grains, like bulgur or brown basmati rice, that may not be available in your local supermarket can often be found in opulent diversity at a natural foods store.

Since whole grains have a shorter shelf life, keep them in the freezer for the best long-term storage when you stock up. That way, you'll always have a good supply when you're inspired to whip up some carbohydrate crowd-pleaser.

Rutabaga with Quatre Epices on Couscous

Flavored with a traditional French spice-pepper blend and served on couscous, this root vegetable takes on an international flair.

 3 cups diced rutabaga
 2 cups water
¼ teaspoon ground cloves
¼ teaspoon ground ginger
¼ teaspoon ground nutmeg
¼ teaspoon white pepper
¼ teaspoon salt
 1 cup whole-wheat couscous (see Note, page 137)
¼ cup golden raisins

Put the rutabaga in a saucepan with the water, cloves, ginger, nutmeg, pepper, and salt. Bring to a simmer, cover, and cook until rutabaga is tender, about 15 minutes. Remove rutabaga with a slotted spoon, and keep it warm.

Measure the cooking liquid, adding enough water to make 2 cups. Bring the broth to a boil in the top of a double boiler over high heat. Reduce heat to medium and gradually add the couscous, and cook, stirring, until the mixture returns to a boil. Place top of double boiler over 1 inch of simmering water, cover, and cook 15 minutes. Uncover and fluff well. Spoon the couscous onto a medium serving platter and break up any remaining clumps. Top with the rutabaga.

Makes 4 servings.

Whole-Wheat Couscous Istanbul

A North African form of pasta, couscous is a precooked wheat product. Package directions for refined couscous, the traditional form that is widely available, call for soaking in a specified amount of hot broth until all the liquid is absorbed. Whole-wheat couscous, available in natural foods stores, contains more of the healthful bran and germ than refined couscous, but it does require some cooking, easily accomplished in a double boiler. Serve this spiced version on the side with any plain poultry dish. Cooked greens make another pleasing accompaniment.

 2 cups Vegetable Stock (page 331), Chicken-Mushroom Stock (page 333), or canned broth
 ¼ teaspoon dried thyme
 ¼ teaspoon ground cumin
 ¼ teaspoon ground cardamom
 ¼ teaspoon ground cinnamon
 ¼ teaspoon anise seeds, crushed
 ¼ cup golden raisins
 2 tablespoons blanched, slivered almonds
 1 cup whole-wheat couscous (see Note, opposite)

Bring the stock to a boil in the top of a double boiler over high heat. Whisk in the thyme, cumin, cardamom, cinnamon, and anise seeds. Stir in the raisins and almonds. Reduce the heat to medium and gradually add the couscous, and cook, stirring, until the mixture returns to a boil.

Place top of double boiler over 1 inch of simmering water, cover, and cook 15 minutes. Uncover and fluff well. Spoon the couscous onto a medium serving platter and break up any remaining clumps.

Makes 4 servings.

VARIATION

Spiced Whole-Wheat Couscous with Apricots

Omit the anise seeds and almonds, and substitute ⅓ cup finely slivered dried apricots for the raisins.

NOTE

If only white refined couscous is available, follow the package directions for cooking. To make 4 servings, you may need about 1½ cups couscous to 2 cups broth.

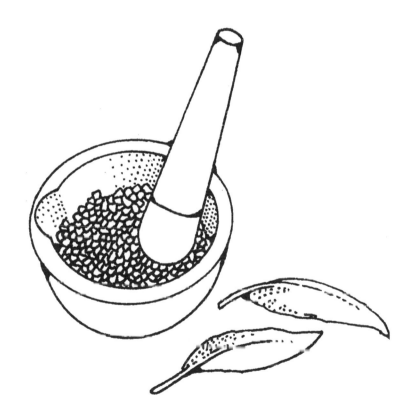

Quinoa with Roasted Squash and Apple

Quinoa (pronounced keen-*wah), a staple of the ancient Inca empire, must always be rinsed before cooking to remove any residue of a natural bitter coating. This version makes a nice side dish with roast chicken.*

¾ pound butternut squash, peeled and diced
1 tablespoon canola oil
½ teaspoon salt
2 Granny Smith apples, peeled, cored, and diced
½ tablespoon butter, cut into pieces
¼ teaspoon ground allspice
   White pepper
¾ cup quinoa
1½ cups water

Preheat the oven to 350F (175C). Toss the squash with the oil and ¼ teaspoon of the salt. Arrange the squash in an 11 × 7-inch baking pan from which you can serve, and bake it 25 minutes. Add the apples and butter; toss again. Bake until the squash and apples are tender, about 15 minutes. Sprinkle with the allspice and white pepper to your taste.

Meanwhile, thoroughly rinse the quinoa in a fine strainer. Combine the quinoa, water, and the remaining ¼ teaspoon salt in a medium saucepan and bring to a boil over medium heat. Reduce the heat to low and simmer, covered, until all the water is absorbed, 12 to 15 minutes, or until the grains turn from white to transparent and the spirallike germ unfurls from the grain.

Gently mix the quinoa with the squash and apples in the baking pan.
Makes 4 servings.

Quinoa Pilaf

Quinoa is so protein-rich that this versatile pilaf could be a vegetarian main dish, with a salad on the side. You could toss in a cup or so of slivered cooked chicken or tiny cooked shrimp for a nonvegetarian main dish, or serve the pilaf as a side dish to the meat or fish course. Anything goes!

1½ cups quinoa
  3 cups Vegetable Stock (page 331), Chicken-Mushroom Stock (page 333), canned broth, or prepared bouillon
 ¼ teaspoon salt (optional)
 ½ cup slivered almonds
  1 tablespoon olive or canola oil
 ½ green bell pepper, seeded and diced
 ½ red bell pepper, seeded and diced
  1 small carrot, very thinly sliced
  1 celery stalk, very thinly sliced
  4 scallions, chopped
  2 tablespoons slivered fresh basil or ½ teaspoon dried
  1 garlic clove, finely minced

Thoroughly rinse the quinoa in a fine strainer. Combine quinoa, stock, and salt, if using, in a medium saucepan and bring to a boil. Reduce the heat and simmer, covered, until all the water is absorbed, 12 to 15 minutes, or until the grains turn from white to transparent and the spirallike germ unfurls from the grain.

Meanwhile, lightly toast the almonds over low heat in a large dry nonstick skillet, only 2 to 3 minutes. Remove the almonds the moment they begin to change color and reserve them.

Heat the oil in the same skillet and sauté the bell peppers, carrot, celery, and scallions until they are lightly colored and crisp-tender, 4 to 5 minutes. Add the basil and garlic, and cook 1 minute. Fluff the quinoa and stir it into the vegetable mixture. Transfer to a serving dish. Sprinkle with almonds.

Makes 4 servings.

Kasha with Cabbage and Egg Noodles

This is a lighter version of a traditional Jewish dish that is prepared with chicken fat and served with sautéed chicken livers. Kasha is always coated with egg and sautéed before cooking, as in the following recipe.

1   cup whole-grain roasted kasha
1   large egg, beaten
3   tablespoons canola oil
2   cups Chicken-Mushroom Stock (page 333) or canned broth
1   large yellow onion, chopped
4   cups finely shredded cabbage
¼   teaspoon salt
1   teaspoon chopped fresh sage or ¼ teaspoon dried
1   teaspoon chopped fresh thyme or ¼ teaspoon dried
     Freshly ground black pepper
8   ounces medium egg noodles, cooked according to package
     directions

In a bowl, toss the kasha with the beaten egg until the grains are completely coated. Heat 1 tablespoon of the oil in a 10-inch skillet over medium heat. Add the kasha and stir-fry over medium heat until all the grains are dry and separate, about 3 minutes. Stir in 1¾ cups of the stock and bring to a simmer. Cover and cook over low heat until the kasha is tender and all the liquid is absorbed, about 15 minutes. Remove from heat and let stand, covered, 10 minutes.

While the kasha is cooking and standing, heat the remaining 2 tablespoons of oil in another large skillet, and sauté the onion until it's softened, 3 to 5 minutes. Add the cabbage, salt, and remaining ¼ cup of the stock. Cover and simmer over low heat until the cabbage is crisp-tender, 3 to 5 minutes. Season the cabbage with the fresh herbs and pepper to taste. Remove the cabbage from the skillet and keep warm.

Drain the noodles. In a large serving dish, toss together the cabbage, kasha, and noodles.

Makes 4 servings.

Oven-Baked Brown and Wild Rice Pilaf

Brown rice and wild rice both need about the same amount of time to cook, so don't substitute white rice in this recipe. Wild rice should be rinsed before cooking.

     1 tablespoon olive or canola oil
    ½ tablespoon butter
     1 medium yellow onion, chopped
     2 celery stalks, chopped
    ¾ cup brown rice
    ¼ cup wild rice, rinsed
     3 cups Vegetable Stock (page 331), Chicken-Mushroom Stock (page 333), or canned broth
    ¼ teaspoon dried thyme
    ¼ teaspoon dried basil
    ¼ teaspoon ground cumin
    ¼ teaspoon salt
    ⅛ teaspoon freshly ground black pepper

Preheat the oven to 375F (190C).

Heat the oil and butter over medium heat in a Dutch oven or other heavy rangetop-to-oven casserole dish with a cover, and sauté the onion and celery until lightly colored, 5 minutes. Add the brown rice and wild rice, stirring to coat with the oil. Stir in the stock, thyme, basil, cumin, salt, and pepper, and bring the mixture to a boil. Cover and bake until all the liquid is absorbed, about 50 minutes. Fluff well before serving.

Makes 6 servings.

Rice Pilaf with Bulgur

In this pilaf, white rice is enriched with whole-grain bulgur, a cracked-wheat product that's available in natural foods stores and some supermarkets.

2 tablespoons canola oil
1 small yellow onion, chopped
1 cup white long-grain rice
½ cup medium bulgur
2¾ cups Vegetable Stock (page 331), Chicken-Mushroom Stock (page 333), or canned broth
¼ cup dried currants
⅛ teaspoon ground cloves
¼ teaspoon salt
Freshly ground black pepper
¼ cup pine nuts, toasted (page 298)
Nonfat plain yogurt, for topping

Heat the oil in a large, heavy saucepan, and sauté the onion until softened, about 5 minutes. Add the rice and stir until all the grains are coated with oil. Add the bulgur, stock, currants, cloves, salt, and pepper to taste. Bring to a boil. Reduce the heat and simmer, covered, until all the liquid is absorbed, about 18 minutes, stirring occasionally to the bottom of the pan with a metal spoon—this pilaf has a tendency to stick.

Spoon the pilaf into a serving dish, and sprinkle it with the pine nuts. Pass a dish of yogurt as a topping.

Makes 6 servings.

Oven-Baked Bulgur Pilaf with Mushrooms

A staple of the Middle East, bulgur has a pleasing nutty flavor that goes well as a side dish with chicken.

  2 tablespoons olive oil
  ¼ cup sliced shallots
  1 small green bell pepper, seeded and diced
  5 ounces button mushrooms, cleaned and sliced
  2 cups Vegetable Stock (page 331), Chicken-Mushroom Stock (page 333), or canned broth
  ¼ teaspoon dried thyme
  ¼ teaspoon salt
  ⅛ teaspoon freshly ground black pepper
  1 cup bulgur

Preheat the oven to 350F (175C).

Heat the oil over medium heat in a Dutch oven or other heavy range-top-to-oven casserole dish with a cover and sauté the shallots, bell pepper, and mushrooms, stirring occasionally, until lightly colored, about 10 minutes. Add the stock, thyme, salt, and pepper, and bring the mixture to a boil. Stir in bulgur. Cover and bake until all the liquid is absorbed, about 25 minutes. Fluff well before serving.

Makes 4 servings.

Brown Basmati Rice

An aromatic rice from India that makes an elegant side dish, whether spiced or plain.

1   cup brown basmati rice (see Note below)
3   cups water
½   teaspoon salt
1   tablespoon canola oil

Rinse the rice. Combine the water, salt, and oil in a medium, heavy saucepan and bring to a boil. Add the rice and reduce the heat until the water is simmering. Cover and cook until all the liquid is absorbed, about 50 minutes. Fluff before serving.
Makes 6 servings.

VARIATION

Spiced Brown Basmati Rice

To the water, add 3 tablespoons fresh lemon juice, ⅓ teaspoon grated lemon peel, ½ teaspoon crushed fennel seeds, and 2 tablespoons coarsely milled flaxseed (optional). When the rice has cooked for 40 minutes, stir in ¼ cup chopped dates and continue cooking until liquid is absorbed.

NOTE
If you substitute refined basmati rice for brown basmati, follow the package directions.

Stir-Fried Brown Rice

This is a basic fried rice that could be enriched with any leftover diced, roasted, or boiled meat. If you do add meat, stir-fry it with the vegetables. Chinese five-spice powder is available with other Asian foods in most supermarkets.

About 2 tablespoons peanut or canola oil
1 egg, beaten with 1 tablespoon water
5 ounces button mushrooms, cleaned and sliced
1 bunch scallions, white parts only, chopped
1 red bell pepper, seeded and cut into small triangles
¼ teaspoon five-spice powder
2 cups cooked brown rice
1 tablespoon naturally brewed soy sauce or to taste

Heat ½ tablespoon of the oil in a large nonstick skillet over medium heat. Pour in egg mixture to form a thin omelet. Cook until set, lifting the edges so that the uncooked portion runs underneath. Remove and reserve the omelet.

Heat the remaining 1½ tablespoons oil in the skillet over medium-high heat and stir-fry the mushrooms, scallions, and bell pepper until they are lightly colored but the pepper is still crisp, 3 to 5 minutes, adding more oil, if needed. Season the vegetables with the five-spice powder. Add the rice. Cut the omelet into thin strips and toss with the rice over low heat to warm all the ingredients. Sprinkle with soy sauce.

Makes 2 main-dish servings.

Orzo and Rice Pilaf

This favorite Armenian dish is traditionally served with calcium-rich yogurt.

2 tablespoons olive oil
¼ cup chopped shallots or green onions
½ cup orzo (rice-shaped pasta)
1 cup Arborio rice or any short-grain white rice
3 cups hot Chicken-Mushroom Stock (page 333) or canned broth
¼ teaspoon dried thyme
¼ teaspoon salt (optional)
   Freshly ground black pepper
1 cup nonfat plain yogurt
2 tablespoons chopped fresh chives

Heat the oil in a deep, heavy saucepan over medium heat and sauté the shallots until they are slightly softened, about 3 minutes. Add the orzo and stir until the grains are golden. Add the rice and stir 1 minute more. Blend in the stock and thyme and salt and pepper to taste. Bring to a boil, stir, and reduce heat until the mixture is just simmering. Cover tightly and simmer over very low heat until the rice is tender and the liquid is absorbed, about 18 minutes. Let stand 5 minutes to absorb any remaining liquid. Fluff well before serving.

Mix the yogurt with the chives, and serve as an accompaniment.
Makes 6 servings.

VARIATION

Orzo and Rice Pilaf with Peas

Prepare the pilaf as above. In a separate pan, cook 1½ cups fresh shelled or frozen green peas in salted water until they are tender, about 5 minutes. Drain and add to the pilaf during its standing time. Stir in 2 tablespoons freshly grated Parmesan cheese. Omit the yogurt and chive accompaniment.

Barley Risotto with Tomatoes

Especially high in soluble fiber, barley is one of the greatest grains for lowering cholesterol, and it's particularly well suited to the requirements of a good risotto—al dente grains napped in a creamy sauce.

 2 tablespoons olive oil
 1 large yellow onion, diced
 1 garlic clove, minced
 1 cup barley, rinsed
 4 cups Chicken-Mushroom Stock (page 333), canned broth, or prepared bouillon
 1 cup peeled, seeded, diced ripe plum tomatoes
 2 tablespoons chopped fresh flat-leaf parsley
¼ cup freshly grated Parmesan cheese
    Freshly ground black pepper

Heat the oil in a large pot over medium heat and sauté the onion and garlic until sizzling and fragrant, about 2 minutes. Add the barley and continue to sauté, stirring, until the grains are coated with oil but not brown, about 2 minutes. Add the stock and tomatoes and bring to a boil. Reduce the heat and simmer over very low heat, with cover slightly ajar, stirring occasionally, until all the liquid is mostly absorbed, about 45 minutes. (If all the liquid is absorbed before the barley is tender, add a little warm water.)

Stir in the parsley, cheese, and pepper. Serve in wide soup bowls as a first course or in a serving bowl as a side dish.

Makes 6 servings.

Virginia's Wild Rice with Mushrooms, Onion, and Cream

My friend Virginia enriches her wild rice with a little cream, which I've found to be a very pleasing indulgence.

1 cup wild rice
4 cups Chicken-Mushroom Stock (page 333) or canned broth
2 tablespoons olive oil
1 small yellow onion, chopped
4 ounces brown mushrooms, cleaned and sliced
   Salt and freshly ground black pepper
2 to 3 tablespoons half-and-half (optional)

Rinse the wild rice in cold water. Bring the stock to a boil, add the wild rice, and simmer, uncovered, until the rice is tender, about 45 minutes. Most of the stock will be absorbed or evaporated. Drain the rice but leave it slightly moist.

While the rice is cooking, heat the oil in a skillet over medium heat and sauté the onion and mushrooms until they are browned, about 8 minutes. Add salt and pepper to taste.

When the rice is almost done, preheat the oven to 325F (165C) and oil a medium casserole dish.

Combine the rice and mushroom mixture in the oiled casserole dish. Stir in the cream. Bake 10 or 15 minutes to heat through and blend flavors.

Makes 4 servings.

Risotto with Shrimp, Peas, and Fresh Herbs

This traditional-style risotto needs careful watching and stirring, so keep the accompanying dishes simple—perhaps a sliced tomato and fennel salad with a loaf of crusty bread.

About 4 cups Vegetable Stock (page 331), Chicken-Mushroom Stock (page 333), or canned broth
1 tablespoon olive oil
1 yellow onion, chopped
1 garlic clove, minced
1½ cups Arborio rice
½ cup dry vermouth, dry white wine, or additional stock
1 cup shelled fresh or frozen peas, thawed to separate
1½ cups cooked, shelled, cleaned small shrimp (page 336)
¼ cup freshly grated Parmesan cheese
1 tablespoon chopped fresh flat-leaf parsley
1 tablespoon chopped fresh chives
1 tablespoon chopped fresh marjoram
Salt and freshly ground black pepper

Bring the stock to a simmer in a medium saucepan and keep it at a simmer.

Meanwhile, heat the oil in a large heavy saucepan over medium heat, and sauté the onion and garlic until softened, 3 minutes. Add the rice and cook, stirring, until all the grains are coated with oil.

Add the vermouth, bring to a boil, and stir often until most of the liquid is absorbed. Add 1 cup of the stock to the rice, and simmer, stirring often, until most of the liquid is absorbed. Add another cup of the hot stock, and simmer, stirring often, until the liquid is almost all absorbed. Continue cooking and adding stock until the rice is almost tender. Add the peas and simmer, adding more stock as needed until the rice is perfectly tender and the mixture is creamy, about 5 more minutes. You may not need all the stock. Stir in the shrimp and heat through, about 2 minutes. Total cooking time is 20 to 30 minutes.

Remove risotto from the heat and stir in the cheese and herbs. Add salt, if needed (the shrimp and cheese are salty), and pepper to taste. Serve immediately.

Makes 4 servings.

Penne Primavera with Asparagus and Peas

Primavera means "spring," and these are the quintessential spring vegetables.

2 tablespoons olive oil
1 bunch scallions, cut diagonally into 1-inch pieces
1 pound fresh asparagus, woody ends trimmed off and spears cut diagonally into 2-inch pieces
1½ cups fresh shelled green peas or 1 (10-oz.) package frozen green peas, thawed to separate
¾ cup Vegetable Stock (page 331), Chicken-Mushroom Stock (page 333), or canned broth
¼ teaspoon salt
Freshly ground black pepper
2 teaspoons minced fresh basil or ½ teaspoon dried
½ teaspoon minced fresh mint or a pinch of dried
8 ounces penne

Heat the oil in a 12-inch skillet, and sauté the scallions over medium heat 2 minutes, or until they just begin to color. Add the asparagus, peas, stock, salt, and pepper to taste and bring to a simmer. Cover and cook until the vegetables are tender, 5 to 8 minutes. Stir in the basil and mint.

Meanwhile, cook the penne according to package directions and drain. In a large serving dish, toss the penne with the vegetables and pan juices.

Makes 2 main-dish servings; 4 first-course or side-dish servings.

Asparagus with Creamy Fettuccine

The creaminess in this sauce comes from nonfat dry milk, not cream.

 1 tablespoon olive oil
 1 small red bell pepper, seeded and diced
 1 garlic clove, minced
 1 pound fresh asparagus, woody stems removed and spears sliced
   diagonally into 1-inch pieces
 ½ cup Vegetable Stock (page 331), Chicken-Mushroom Stock
   (page 333), or canned broth
 3 tablespoons nonfat dry milk
 2 tablespoons instant flour, such as Wondra
 ¼ teaspoon salt
 ¼ teaspoon white pepper
 1½ cups low-fat or whole milk
 8 ounces fresh or dried fettuccine
 ⅓ cup freshly grated Parmesan cheese

Heat the oil in a 12-inch skillet over medium heat, and sauté the bell pepper, stirring often, until crisp-tender, 3 to 5 minutes. Add the garlic and cook 1 minute. Remove and reserve the bell pepper and any garlic that clings to it.

Add the asparagus and stock to the skillet and bring to a simmer. Cover and cook until crisp-tender, 3 to 5 minutes. Remove the asparagus with a slotted spoon, leaving the juices in the pan; reserve asparagus.

Whisk the dry milk, flour, salt, and pepper into the liquid milk. Stir mixture into the pan juices, and cook over medium heat, stirring constantly, until bubbling and thick. Reduce heat and simmer, stirring constantly, 3 minutes. Return the bell pepper and asparagus to the pan, and stir to combine. Keep warm.

Cook the fettuccine according to the package directions and drain. In a large serving dish, toss the fettuccine with the asparagus mixture. Add the cheese and toss again. Serve immediately.

Makes 2 main-dish servings; 4 first-course or side-dish servings.

Broccoli with Portobello Mushrooms and Rigatoni

The superstar of vegetables, broccoli adds nutrients, crunch, and color to this dish.

  1 bunch (about 1 lb.) broccoli
 10 ounces Portobello mushrooms, cleaned
     About 2 tablespoons olive oil, or more as needed
  1 to 2 garlic cloves, minced
  2 cups peeled, seeded, chopped fresh tomatoes, or 1 (14- to 16-oz.)
     can tomatoes, chopped
  2 tablespoons minced fresh flat-leaf parsley
 ¼ teaspoon salt
 ⅛ teaspoon freshly ground black pepper
 ⅛ teaspoon hot red pepper flakes
 12 ounces rigatoni
     Freshly grated Parmesan cheese, to pass

Separate the broccoli into stalks and flowerets. Cut the stalks into 1-inch pieces. Cook the broccoli flowerets in boiling salted water until crisp-tender, about 3 minutes. Remove with a slotted spoon and immediately rinse with cool water to stop the cooking action. Cook the stalk pieces in the same water until tender, about 5 minutes. Drain and rinse. Combine stalks and flowerets.

If the Portobellos are button-size, just cut off the bottom of each stem and leave them whole. Otherwise, cut them into ½-inch-wide slices.

Heat the oil in a 10-inch nonstick skillet over medium-high heat, and sauté the mushrooms, stirring often, until they begin to brown, 3 minutes. Add the garlic and cook 1 minute. Add the tomatoes and cook until they are slightly softened, 5 minutes. Stir in the broccoli, parsley, salt, black pepper, and pepper flakes.

Meanwhile, cook the rigatoni according to package directions and drain. Toss the rigatoni with the broccoli mixture in a large serving dish. Pass grated cheese at the table.

Makes 4 servings.

Broccoli and Summer Squash with Penne

Choose broccoli flowerets with tightly closed buds and a deep green color for the best flavor.

¾ pound broccoli flowerets, cut into uniform pieces
1 medium summer squash, sliced into half-rounds
   About 2 tablespoons olive oil
4 ounces mushrooms, cleaned and sliced
1 small red bell pepper, seeded and diced
1 garlic clove, minced
   Salt and freshly ground black pepper
8 ounces penne
3 tablespoons freshly grated Parmesan cheese

Cook the broccoli in a large pot of boiling salted water until crisp-tender, about 3 minutes. Remove with a slotted spoon. Cook the summer squash in the same water until tender, about 2 minutes. Drain, reserving ½ cup of the cooking water.

Heat the oil in a large nonstick skillet and sauté the mushrooms over medium heat, stirring often, until their juices evaporate and they begin to brown. Add the bell pepper and cook until the bell pepper is softened, 3 minutes, adding more oil, if needed. Add the garlic and cook 1 minute. Add the broccoli and summer squash, and heat through to blend flavors. Season the vegetables with salt and pepper.

Meanwhile cook the penne according to package directions. Toss the penne with the vegetables and reserved cooking water in a large serving dish. Sprinkle with cheese and serve.

Makes 2 main-dish servings; 4 first-course or side-dish servings.

Broccoli Rabe with Zucchini and Shells

Two great things about zucchini: It doesn't sponge up oil (unlike egg-plant) and it sweetens as it sautés, complementing the sharp taste of rabe.

 1 bunch (about ¾ lb.) broccoli rabe (rapini)
 2 tablespoons olive oil
 1 medium zucchini, cut crosswise into 1-inch-thick chunks
 2 garlic cloves, finely chopped
 1 cup Vegetable Stock (page 331), Chicken-Mushroom Stock (page 333), or canned broth
 4 oil-packed, sun-dried tomatoes, drained and chopped
 1 tablespoon chopped fresh basil or 1 teaspoon dried
 ¼ teaspoon salt
   Freshly ground black pepper
12 ounces medium pasta shells
 3 tablespoons freshly grated Romano cheese, plus more to pass

Wash the rabe well. Trim off the tough stem ends and chop the rabe coarsely.

Heat the oil in a 12-inch skillet over medium heat and stir-fry the zucchini until it begins to brown and is tender, 5 minutes. Add the garlic and cook 1 minute. Remove the zucchini with a slotted spoon; reserve.

Add the stock, tomatoes, and rabe to the skillet. Cover and simmer until the rabe is tender, about 10 minutes. Season it with basil, salt, and pepper. Return the zucchini to the pan and heat through.

Cook the pasta according to package directions and drain. Combine the pasta and vegetable mixture in a large serving dish and toss with cheese. Pass more cheese at the table.

Makes 4 servings.

Broccoli Rabe with Roasted Peppers and Gemelli

Also called rapini, this popular Italian vegetable has a slight bitterness that combines well with sweet bell peppers.

2 red bell peppers (see Note below)
1 bunch (about ¾ lb.) broccoli rabe
2 tablespoons olive oil
1 garlic clove, minced
   About ½ cup chicken broth or water
   Salt and freshly ground black pepper
   Dashes of hot red pepper flakes (optional)
12 ounces gemelli or rotelle

Preheat the broiler. Roast the bell peppers about 4 inches below the heat source, using tongs to turn them often, until sides are blistered and charred and the peppers are tender, about 10 minutes. When pressed with the back of a cooking fork, they should collapse a little. Put the bell peppers in a covered casserole. When they are cool enough to handle, seed and peel the peppers and cut them into strips.

Trim off the tough stem ends and chop the rabe into 2-inch pieces. Heat the oil in a large pot over medium heat and sauté the garlic until sizzling, 1 minute. Add the rabe and broth, cover, and cook until the rabe is tender, about 10 minutes, adding more broth, if necessary. There should be about ¼ cup liquid, enough to keep the rabe juicy. Combine the rabe and bell peppers; heat through.

Cook the pasta according to package directions and drain. Toss the pasta with the rabe in a serving dish.

Makes 4 servings.

NOTE
You can substitute an 8-ounce jar of Italian roasted peppers for the fresh bell peppers.

Vermicelli with Roasted Garlic, Walnuts, and Fresh Herbs

Roasting the garlic bulb is one way to get lots of immunity-boosting garlic with a mellow flavor rather than a strong garlicky taste.

 1 garlic bulb
⅓ cup extra-virgin olive oil
½ cup walnut halves
¼ teaspoon hot red pepper flakes
⅓ cup warm chicken or vegetable broth
12 ounces vermicelli, cooked according to package directions
½ cup finely chopped fresh flat-leaf parsley
¼ cup finely chopped fresh basil or a combination of basil
   and marjoram
   Freshly grated Romano cheese, to pass

Preheat the oven to 375F (190C). Cut off the top of the garlic bulb and wrap the bulb in foil. Bake 45 minutes or until fragrant and soft when pressed. Let the garlic cool enough to handle. Squeeze the garlic cloves out of their peels.

Heat the oil in a small skillet over very low heat and stir in the garlic, breaking it up with the back of a spoon. Add the walnuts and heat 1 minute. Add the pepper flakes and broth.

Drain the vermicelli. Toss with the garlic-walnut mixture and the fresh herbs. Pass the cheese at the table.

Makes 2 main-dish servings; 4 first-course or side-dish servings.

Cannellini, Fennel, and Red Bell Pepper with Linguine

A delicious ten-minute pasta sauce for the after-work gourmet. Rub the cut side of leftover fresh fennel with lemon or vinegar and wrap in foil to help prevent browning.

2   tablespoons olive oil
1   large red bell pepper, seeded and diced
1   cup diced fennel
2   garlic cloves, minced
1   (14- to 16-oz.) can cannellini (white kidney beans), drained and rinsed, or 2 cups cooked (page 328)
1   cup Vegetable Stock (page 331), Chicken-Mushroom Stock (page 333), or canned broth
1   tablespoon chopped fresh summer savory or 1 teaspoon dried
¼   teaspoon salt
    Freshly ground black pepper
    Hot red pepper flakes
2   tablespoons finely chopped fresh flat-leaf parsley
12 ounces linguine
    Freshly grated Parmesan cheese

Heat the oil in a large skillet over medium heat and sauté the bell pepper and fennel until tender and lightly browned, 5 to 7 minutes. Add the garlic and cook 1 minute. Add the beans, stock, savory, salt, black pepper, and pepper flakes to taste. Simmer 5 minutes. Add the parsley and remove from the heat.

Cook the linguine according to package directions and drain. Toss the linguine with the bean sauce in a large serving dish. Pass grated cheese at the table.

Makes 2 main-dish servings; 4 first course or side-dish servings.

Braised Zucchini, Green Beans, and Mushrooms with Rigatoni

Chunky rigatoni complements a chunky vegetable sauce.

 2 tablespoons olive oil
10 ounces button mushrooms, cleaned and halved
 1 medium zucchini, cut crosswise into 1-inch-thick chunks
½ pound fresh green beans, trimmed and cut into 2-inch lengths
 1 green bell pepper, seeded and cut into 1-inch chunks
½ teaspoon dried oregano
   Salt and freshly ground black pepper
 2 garlic cloves, minced
 6 oil-packed, sun-dried tomatoes, drained and slivered
½ cup chicken broth
12 ounces rigatoni
¼ cup freshly grated Romano cheese

Heat the oil in a Dutch oven or deep, heavy pot over medium-high heat and sauté the mushrooms, stirring occasionally until their juices evaporate and they begin to brown. Add the zucchini, green beans, and bell pepper. Braise over medium heat, stirring often, until the zucchini is golden and the beans are crisp-tender, about 5 minutes. Add the oregano and salt and pepper to taste. Add the garlic and sauté 1 minute. Add the tomatoes and stock; cook 1 minute more.

Cook the rigatoni according to package directions and drain. Toss the vegetables with the pasta and cheese in a large serving dish.

Makes 4 servings.

Cauliflower and Brown Mushrooms
with Fresh Linguine

Instead of serving ricotta-stuffed pasta, Italian families sometimes simply pass a bowl of ricotta to be spooned on as desired.

 1 cup part-skim ricotta cheese
½ cup freshly grated Romano cheese
 1 medium head cauliflower, trimmed and separated into flowerets
 2 tablespoons olive oil
10 ounces brown mushrooms, cleaned and sliced
 1 large garlic clove, minced
 2 tablespoons chopped fresh flat-leaf parsley
¼ teaspoon hot red pepper flakes
¼ teaspoon salt
12 ounces fresh linguine

Mix the ricotta and Romano cheese and set aside. Cook the cauliflower in boiling salted water until crisp-tender, about 3 minutes. Drain, reserving ½ cup of the cooking water.

Heat the oil in a 12-inch nonstick skillet over medium heat and sauté the mushrooms, stirring often, until the moisture evaporates and they turn brown, about 5 minutes. Add the garlic and cook 1 minute. Add the cauliflower, parsley, pepper flakes, and salt and toss the mixture lightly. Add enough of the reserved cooking water to make the mixture slightly moist.

Cook the linguine according to package directions and drain. Toss the linguine with the cauliflower in a serving dish. Pass the ricotta mixture separately to be spooned on top.

Makes 4 servings.

Peas and Prosciutto with Spaghetti

Just a little ham adds a lot of flavor—when it's prosciutto.

6 thin slices (about ⅛ lb.) prosciutto
1 small yellow onion, chopped
1 garlic clove, chopped
1 (3-inch) piece of celery, chopped
1 tablespoon olive oil
2 cups fresh shelled or frozen green peas, thawed to separate
1 large ripe tomato, peeled, seeded, and chopped
½ cup chicken broth
1 tablespoon chopped fresh flat-leaf parsley
1 tablespoon chopped fresh basil or ½ teaspoon dried
¼ teaspoon salt
  Freshly ground black pepper
8 ounces spaghetti
1 tablespoon unsalted butter, cut into pieces
  Grated Parmesan cheese, to pass

With a chef's knife, on a cutting board, mince the prosciutto, onion, garlic, and celery. Heat the oil in a large skillet over low heat. Add the onion mixture and slowly sauté until it's lightly colored, about 5 minutes. Add the peas, tomato, and broth. Cover and simmer until the peas are tender, 5 to 8 minutes. Season with parsley, basil, salt, and pepper to taste.

Cook the spaghetti according to package directions and drain. Toss it with the butter in a large serving bowl. Add the peas mixture and toss again. Pass cheese at the table.

Makes 2 main-dish servings; 4 first-course or side-dish servings.

Spinach, Pine Nuts, and Feta with Ziti

This pasta dish was inspired by Greek cuisine.

- 1 pound fresh young spinach
- 3 tablespoons olive oil
- 1 yellow onion chopped
- 3 garlic cloves, finely chopped
- ½ teaspoon salt
- ¼ teaspoon black pepper
- ⅛ teaspoon hot red pepper flakes, or more, to your taste
- 12 ounces ziti or penne
- 4 ounces feta cheese, crumbled
- ⅓ cup pine nuts, lightly toasted (page 298)

Wash the spinach well and remove any tough stems. Chop it coarsely. Heat the oil in a large pot over medium heat and sauté the onion until lightly colored, 3 to 5 minutes. Add the garlic and cook 1 minute. Add the spinach with just the moisture that clings to its leaves after washing, cover pot, and steam over low heat until it has wilted, about 3 minutes. Season with salt, black pepper, and pepper flakes.

Cook the pasta according to package directions and drain. If necessary, reheat the spinach mixture. Toss the pasta, feta, and spinach together in a large serving dish. Sprinkle with pine nuts.

Makes 2 main-dish servings; 4 first-course or side-dish servings.

Escarole Sicilian with Linguine

This pasta dish from Sicily is an especially delicious combination of flavors.

1 big bunch (1 lb.) escarole
3 tablespoons olive oil
4 anchovy fillets (optional), chopped
1 garlic clove, minced or pressed through a garlic press
1 cup Vegetable Stock (page 331), Chicken-Mushroom Stock (page 333), or canned broth
3 tablespoons golden raisins
   Salt and freshly ground black pepper
½ cup pitted Sicilian ripe olives, halved
12 ounces fresh or dry linguine
¼ cup pine nuts, lightly toasted (page 298)
   Freshly grated Parmesan cheese, to pass
   Hot red pepper flakes, to pass

Wash the escarole well. Hold the bunch together and cut it crosswise into thirds.

Heat the oil in a 12-inch skillet over very low heat and sauté the anchovies, if using, until they begin to soften. Add the garlic and cook 1 minute. Add the escarole, stock, and raisins. Cover and simmer until the escarole is just tender, about 10 minutes. Season with salt (less if using the anchovies) and pepper to taste. Stir in the olives.

Cook the pasta according to package directions and drain. Toss it with the escarole in a large serving dish. Sprinkle the pine nuts on top. Pass the grated cheese and pepper flakes at the table.

Makes 2 main-dish servings; 4 first-course or side-dish servings.

Sweet Potatoes and Gorgonzola with Shells

A little Gorgonzola cheese goes a long way in flavoring this simple dish. Sweet potatoes are especially rich in beta-carotene.

2   large sweet potatoes, peeled and diced
2   tablespoons olive oil
2   garlic cloves, minced
1   teaspoon chopped fresh thyme leaves or ¼ teaspoon dried
¼   teaspoon salt
⅛   teaspoon freshly ground black pepper
8   ounces medium pasta shells
      About 1 cup warmed Vegetable Stock (page 331), Chicken-Mushroom Stock (page 333), or canned broth
2   ounces (about ⅓ cup) crumbled Gorgonzola cheese, at room temperature

Cook the sweet potatoes in boiling salted water until tender, about 5 minutes; drain. Heat the oil in a large skillet over medium heat and sauté the garlic until it's sizzling and fragrant, about 2 minutes. Add the sweet potatoes, thyme, salt, and pepper, and stir-fry 3 minutes to blend flavors.

Cook the shells according to package directions and drain. Toss them gently with the sweet potato mixture and enough broth to moisten. Add the cheese, and toss again.

Makes 2 main-dish servings; 4 first-course or side-dish servings.

Sautéed Scallops and Peas with Linguine

Tiny bay scallops are very sweet and succulent.

 1 pound bay scallops
    All-purpose flour, for dusting
 2 tablespoons olive oil
 1 garlic clove, minced
 2 tablespoons fresh lemon juice
 1 tablespoon minced fresh flat-leaf parsley
 ¼ teaspoon salt
    Freshly ground black pepper
 2 cups shelled fresh or frozen green peas
 ½ cup chicken broth
    Several leaves of fresh basil, slivered
 1 red bell pepper, roasted, peeled (page 155), and diced (see Note
    below)
12 ounces fresh or dried linguine

Rinse and drain the scallops. Dust them with flour. Heat the oil in a 12-inch skillet over high heat and stir-fry the scallops until they are lightly colored and cooked through, 3 to 5 minutes. Add the garlic during the last minute. Season with lemon juice, parsley, salt, and black pepper.

Boil the peas in the broth in a saucepan until tender, 5 to 8 minutes; do not drain. Season with basil and black pepper. Add the roasted pepper.

Cook the linguine according to package directions and drain. Toss it with the scallops and vegetables and serve at once.

Makes 4 servings.

NOTE

You can use a large roasted bell pepper from a jar instead of roasting a fresh bell pepper.

Lemony Shrimp and Crabmeat with Vermicelli

An easy, elegant, and surprisingly light first course or main dish. Once upon a time, this dish would have been drenched in heavy cream.

1½ cups low-fat or whole milk
 ¼ cup nonfat dry milk
 3 tablespoons instant flour, such as Wondra
 ¼ teaspoon dried tarragon
 ¼ teaspoon salt
 ⅛ teaspoon ground turmeric
 ⅛ teaspoon white pepper
    Cayenne pepper
 ¼ teaspoon grated lemon peel
    Juice of ½ lemon (about 2 tablespoons)
 6 ounces cooked, shelled, deveined shrimp (page 336)
 1 (3- to 4-oz.) can crabmeat, drained, rinsed, and flaked
 8 ounces vermicelli
 2 tablespoons finely chopped fresh flat-leaf parsley

Combine the liquid milk, dry milk, flour, tarragon, salt, turmeric, white pepper, and cayenne to taste in a heavy saucepan and whisk until smooth. Cook over medium heat, stirring constantly, until the sauce bubbles and thickens; this sauce will stick easily, so stir and watch carefully.

Stir in the lemon peel and lemon juice, and simmer 2 minutes. Add the shrimp and crabmeat, and warm them in the sauce 5 to 10 minutes to develop the flavor.

Cook the vermicelli according to package directions and drain. Spoon it into a large serving dish and top with the sauce. Sprinkle with parsley.

Makes 2 main-dish servings; 4 first-course servings.

Skillet Bolognese Sauce with Shells

*A traditional meat sauce made lighter by using lean ground turkey
(stretched with zucchini) instead of beef.*

About 2 tablespoons olive oil
1 pound lean ground turkey
1 medium zucchini, quartered lengthwise and cut crosswise into
    1-inch-thick chunks
1 red bell pepper, seeded and cut into 1-inch chunks
1 garlic clove, minced
1 dried hot red chile
1 (28-oz.) can Italian plum tomatoes with juice (not puree)
½ cup dry white vermouth or dry white wine (optional)
¼ teaspoon fennel seeds
½ teaspoon salt
¼ teaspoon freshly ground black pepper
12 ounces medium pasta shells
1 tablespoon minced fresh flat-leaf parsley
6 leaves of fresh basil, chopped, or ½ teaspoon dried
2 tablespoons freshly grated Romano cheese, plus more to pass

Heat the oil in a 12-inch skillet over medium heat and brown the
ground meat, breaking it up as it cooks. Remove the meat with a slotted
spoon and set aside. Adding more oil if needed, sauté the zucchini and
red bell pepper 5 minutes. Add the garlic and chile and cook 1 minute,
stirring. Add the tomatoes, vermouth, if using, fennel seeds, salt, black
pepper, and reserved meat. Cook over medium-high heat, stirring often,
20 minutes.

Meanwhile, cook the shells according to package directions until al
dente and drain pasta. Remove the chile from sauce and add the
pasta. Stir in the parsley and basil. Cook over low heat 2 to 3 minutes
to develop the flavor. Stir in the cheese, and pass more at the table.

Makes 4 servings.

VARIATION

Skillet Bolognese Sauce with Chick-Peas

Follow the preceding recipe, substituting 1 cup cooked chick-peas (page 328) or 1 (8.5-oz.) can chick-peas, drained and rinsed, for the zucchini.

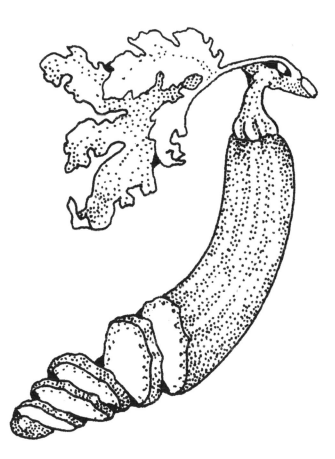

Roasted Vegetable and Pasta Salad

Roasting the vegetables brings out their richest flavor.

3 tablespoons olive oil
4 baby or Japanese eggplant, unpeeled, halved lengthwise
2 small zucchini, halved lengthwise
4 plum tomatoes, halved
2 red bell peppers. seeded and cut into chunks
4 garlic cloves, peeled and crushed
1 tablespoon chopped fresh marjoram or 1 teaspoon dried oregano
   Salt
8 ounces penne
2 tablespoons red wine vinegar
2 tablespoons chopped fresh flat-leaf parsley
   Freshly ground black pepper

Preheat the oven to 375F (190C). Pour 2 tablespoons of oil into a large roasting pan that will hold the vegetables snugly in one layer. Add the vegetables and stir to coat all sides with oil. Arrange the eggplant, zucchini, and tomatoes cut sides up. Sprinkle with marjoram and ¼ teaspoon salt. Bake on the middle rack 45 minutes to 1 hour, or until the vegetables are very tender. Check halfway through the cooking time; remove the garlic if it's getting too brown. Let the vegetables cool until they can be handled. Mince the garlic; dice the other vegetables.

Cook the penne according to package directions, drain, and rinse in cold water. In a large bowl, toss the vegetables and penne with the vinegar, the remaining 1 tablespoon of oil, parsley, salt, and pepper. Taste to see if you want more oil or vinegar. Serve at room temperature.

Makes 4 servings.

Date-Nut Muffins

Whole-grain goodness in the milled flaxseed and oats makes these muffins as good for you as they are tasty. You can start preparing the muffins the night before baking; mix together and refrigerate the liquid ingredients and stir together the dry ingredients. Blend the two mixtures the next morning just before spooning the batter into the muffin cups.

1½ cups unbleached all-purpose flour
  1 tablespoon baking powder
  ½ teaspoon ground cinnamon
  ½ teaspoon salt
  ¾ cup quick-cooking oatmeal
  ¼ cup milled flaxseed (available in natural foods stores)
  1 cup chopped pitted dates
  ½ cup chopped walnuts
  ¾ cup milk
  2 large eggs or ½ cup egg substitute
  ⅓ cup canola oil
  ½ cup packed dark brown sugar

Preheat the oven to 400F (205C). Spray a 12-cup nonstick muffin pan with nonstick cooking spray, or use paper liners.

Sift together the flour, baking powder, cinnamon, and salt into a bowl. Stir in the oats, flaxseed, dates, and walnuts.

In a separate bowl, beat together the milk, eggs, oil, and brown sugar until blended.

Pour the liquid ingredients into the dry ingredients and mix just to blend. Divide the batter among the muffin cups.

Place the muffin pan on the top rack, and immediately decrease the oven temperature to 375F (190C). Bake about 18 minutes, until the muffins are golden brown and a wooden pick inserted in the center of a muffin comes out clean.

Carefully remove muffins from the pan and transfer to a wire rack. Serve warm or at room temperature.

Makes 12 muffins.

Blueberry Muffins

"Real" homemade muffins, unlike bakery cake muffins, are not heavily sugared. In this batch, most of the butter has been replaced with canola oil.

2½ cups unbleached all-purpose flour
 ½ cup sugar
2¼ teaspoons baking powder
 ½ teaspoon salt
 ¼ teaspoon ground cinnamon
 1 cup whole or low-fat milk
 2 large eggs or ½ cup egg substitute
 ⅓ cup canola oil
 2 tablespoons butter, melted and cooled
 1 heaping cup blueberries, preferably small blueberries
   Cinnamon Sugar (page 338)

Preheat the oven to 400F (205C). Spray a 12-cup nonstick muffin pan with nonstick cooking spray, or use paper liners.

Sift together the flour, sugar, baking powder, salt, and cinnamon into a large bowl.

In a separate bowl, beat together the milk, eggs, oil, and butter.

Pour the liquid ingredients into the dry ingredients, and mix just to blend. Fold in the blueberries. Divide the batter among the muffin cups, and sprinkle them with cinnamon sugar.

Bake in the top third of the oven 15 to 18 minutes, until the muffins are golden brown and the blueberries on top have broken open, yielding trails of blue juice.

Carefully remove muffins from the pan and transfer to a wire rack. Serve warm or at room temperature.

Makes 12 muffins.

VARIATION

Cranberry Muffins

Substitute ground cardamom for the cinnamon, increase the sugar to ⅔ cup, and use 1½ cups chopped fresh cranberries in place of blueberries. Omit cinnamon sugar.

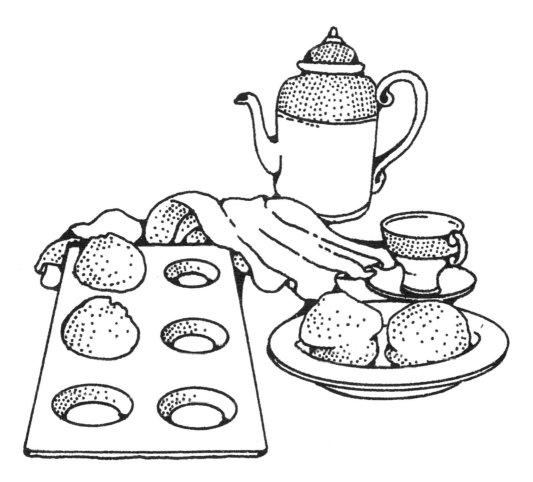

Squash Baking Powder Biscuits

The squash adds a golden color along with some beta-carotene to these biscuits.

2½ cups unbleached all-purpose flour
 2 tablespoons light brown sugar
 1 tablespoon baking powder
 ½ teaspoon salt
 ¼ teaspoon ground allspice
 2 tablespoons unsalted butter, chilled
 ⅓ cup canola oil
 ¾ cup mashed cooked butternut squash
   About ½ cup whole or low-fat milk

Preheat the oven to 400F (205C). Spray a baking sheet with nonstick cooking spray.

Sift together the flour, brown sugar, baking powder, salt, and allspice into a bowl. Use a pastry cutter or 2 knives to cut the butter into the flour until it forms granules the size of small peas. Whisk together the oil and squash, and stir it into the flour mixture. Blend carefully; the mixture will be very thick. Add enough milk to make a soft dough.

Transfer the dough to a floured surface, and knead it gently until it can be patted into a ½-inch-thick round. With a floured biscuit cutter or glass, cut the biscuits and place them on the baking sheet, rerolling scraps.

Bake the biscuits on the top rack about 12 minutes, or until the tops are lightly browned and firm. Serve warm.

Makes about 12 biscuits.

Blueberry Double-Corn Bread

The flavors of late summer! Try this for a super brunch bread or as the accompaniment to a relaxed chowder supper.

½ tablespoon butter
1 cup finely ground cornmeal, preferably whole-grain
1 cup unbleached all-purpose flour
2 tablespoons sugar
1 tablespoon baking powder
½ teaspoon salt
⅛ teaspoon ground nutmeg
1 cup whole or low-fat milk
1 large egg
¼ cup canola oil
  About ¾ cup fresh corn kernels or frozen whole-kernel corn, thawed
¾ cup fresh or frozen blueberries

Preheat the oven to 375F (190C) and melt butter in a 9- to 10-inch cast-iron skillet or a 9-inch-square baking pan. Brush the butter over the bottom and sides of the skillet. This will give a "buttery" taste to the crust even though only unsaturated vegetable oil is used in the bread itself.

Sift together the cornmeal, flour, sugar, baking powder, salt, and nutmeg into a bowl.

In a separate bowl, beat together the milk, egg, and oil. Pour the liquid ingredients into the dry ingredients and mix just to blend. Fold in the corn and blueberries.

Bake in the top third of the oven 25 minutes or until the crust is golden brown and a wooden pick inserted near the center comes out clean. Let cool slightly. Cut into wedges to serve.

Makes 8 servings.

Apricot Tea Bread

A low-fat fruit-and-nut-studded tea treat that slices and keeps well—and it's rich in antioxidant vitamins!

½ cup orange juice
1 cup diced dried apricots (see Note opposite)
½ cup chopped pitted dates
2½ cups unbleached all-purpose flour
2½ teaspoons baking powder
½ teaspoon baking soda
½ teaspoon salt
¼ teaspoon ground ginger
¼ teaspoon ground cinnamon
¼ teaspoon ground nutmeg
2 eggs or ½ cup egg substitute
½ cup packed dark brown sugar
½ cup buttermilk or sour milk (page 338)
¼ cup canola oil
¾ cup chopped walnuts

Preheat the oven to 350F (175C). Spray a 9 × 5-inch loaf pan with nonstick cooking spray and line the bottom with wax paper.

Heat the orange juice to boiling in a small saucepan. Stir in the apricots and dates. Remove pan from the heat, and let the mixture stand until needed.

Sift together the flour, baking powder, soda, salt, and spices into a bowl.

In the bowl of an electric mixer or, by hand, in a separate large bowl, beat together the eggs, sugar, buttermilk, and oil until blended. Add the dry ingredients and beat until combined. Stir in the apricot mixture. Fold in the nuts. Spoon the batter into the prepared pan.

Bake on the middle rack about 50 minutes or until the bread has risen, browned, split, and the split appears dry, then test with a wooden pick or cake tester. The bread is done when the wooden pick comes out clean.

Let the bread cool in the pan on a wire rack 5 minutes. Turn out the bread and peel off the wax paper. Cool completely on wire rack. Wrap well in foil for storage.

Makes 1 loaf, 8 to 10 slices.

NOTE

To dice dried apricots or other dried fruit, snip them with kitchen shears.

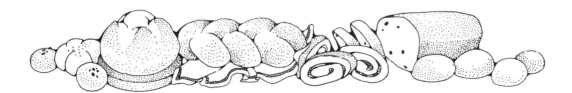

Walnut-Cinnamon Coffeecake with Flaxseed

Using flaxseed in baking is an easy way to add omega-3 fatty acids to your diet.

½ cup chopped walnuts
⅓ cup packed dark brown sugar
1 teaspoon ground cinnamon
2¼ cups unbleached all-purpose flour
¾ cup granulated sugar
2 teaspoons baking powder
½ teaspoon baking soda
¼ teaspoon salt
⅓ cup milled flaxseed
1 cup buttermilk or sour milk (page 338)
½ cup canola oil
2 large eggs, beaten
2 teaspoons vanilla extract
½ cup raisins, plumped in hot water and drained

Preheat the oven to 350F (175C). Spray a medium tube pan with a removable rim with nonstick cooking spray, or butter and flour it.

Mix together the walnuts, brown sugar, and cinnamon and set aside.

Sift together the flour, granulated sugar, baking powder, soda, and salt in a large bowl. Stir in the milled flaxseed.

In the bowl of an electric mixer or, by hand, in another large bowl, beat together the buttermilk, oil, eggs, and vanilla. Add the flour mixture, and beat until blended. Stir in the raisins.

Spoon half the batter into the prepared pan. Sprinkle with half the reserved walnut mixture. Spread the remaining batter on top. Sprinkle with the remaining walnut mixture.

Bake on the middle rack until a wooden pick or cake tester inserted in the center comes out dry, about 45 minutes. Cool in the pan on a wire rack 5 minutes. Remove the rim. When the coffeecake is completely cool, remove it from the rest of the pan.

Makes 12 servings.

Corn and Scallion Griddle Cakes

These savory cakes can be served as a luncheon dish or as a side dish at dinner.

  2 cups fresh corn kernels or frozen whole-kernel corn
  4 scallions, with green tops, finely chopped
  1 cup unbleached all-purpose flour
  1 teaspoon baking powder
  ½ teaspoon salt
  ⅛ teaspoon cayenne pepper
  ¼ cup toasted wheat germ
  ¾ cup low-fat or whole milk
  1 large egg, beaten, or ¼ cup egg substitute
  2 tablespoons canola oil
     Zesty Fresh Tomato Salsa (page 330) or other salsa as an
     accompaniment (optional)

Combine the corn and scallions in a saucepan with water to cover, bring to a boil, and cook 5 minutes, or until the corn is tender. Drain and cool the vegetables.

Sift together the flour, baking powder, salt, and cayenne into a large bowl. Stir in the wheat germ.

Whisk the milk and egg with 1 tablespoon of the oil in a small bowl. Pour the liquid ingredients into the dry, stirring to blend. Fold in the corn and scallions.

Use some of the remaining tablespoon of oil to coat a nonstick 12-inch skillet, and heat it over medium-low heat. Drop the batter by ¼ cupfuls onto the hot skillet. Cook until bubbles form on the tops and the bottoms are golden, 2 to 3 minutes. Turn and cook until the second sides are golden. Keep cooked cakes warm while cooking a second batch. Brush the pan with more oil as needed. If the batter gets too thick, add a little more milk.

Serve cakes warm. Pass salsa at the table, if using.

Makes 12 cakes; 4 servings.

Pumpkin Pancakes

Compared to, say, a Danish pastry or a doughnut, pancakes are one of the least fatty of breakfast sweets.

1¾ cups unbleached all-purpose flour
1½ teaspoons baking powder
 ½ teaspoon baking soda
 ½ teaspoon salt
 ¼ teaspoon ground cinnamon
 ¼ teaspoon ground ginger
 ⅛ teaspoon ground cloves
 ¼ cup wheat germ
1⅔ cups buttermilk or sour milk (page 338)
 ¾ cup cooked, mashed pumpkin or solid pack unflavored canned
    pumpkin (see Note opposite)
 ½ cup packed light brown sugar
 2 large eggs or ½ cup egg substitute
 2 tablespoons butter, melted, plus more for cooking
    Pure maple syrup, for topping

Sift together the flour, baking powder, soda, salt, and spices into a large bowl. Stir in the wheat germ.

In another bowl or a food processor, blend together the buttermilk, pumpkin, sugar, eggs, and butter until smooth. Pour the pumpkin mixture into the dry ingredients, and whisk to blend.

Heat a nonstick electric grill to 400F (205C) or heat a large nonstick frying pan over medium heat until hot. Brush lightly with melted butter, and drop the batter by ¼ cupfuls onto the hot surface. Cook until bubbles form on the tops and the bottoms are golden, 2 to 3 minutes. Turn and cook until the second sides are golden. Keep the cooked cakes warm while baking the rest in batches.

Serve with maple syrup.

Makes 16 to 18 cakes; 4 servings.

NOTE

Leftovers from an opened can of pumpkin can be frozen for later use. They do become a bit watery when thawed, but you can simply drain off the colorless liquid and use the rest.

Irish Brown Bread

A quick whole-grain bread is crumbly and satisfying, enriched with extra wheat germ and sweetened with dried currants.

  1 cup dried currants or raisins
  2 cups whole-wheat flour
     cups unbleached all-purpose flour
 ¼ cup sugar
  1 tablespoon baking soda
  1 teaspoon salt
 ¼ cup toasted wheat germ
 ½ teaspoon caraway seeds (optional)
 ¼ teaspoon freshly ground nutmeg or allspice (optional)
 ¼ cup canola oil
  2 to 2½ cups buttermilk or sour milk (page 338)

Preheat the oven to 350F (175C). Spray 2 (9-inch-round) pans with nonstick cooking spray.

Soak the currants in very hot water 5 minutes to plump them; drain.

Stir together the flours, sugar, soda, and salt in a large bowl. Stir in the wheat germ, currants, caraway seeds, and nutmeg, if using. Add oil and enough buttermilk to make a soft but manageable dough. Knead the dough briefly in the bowl, and form it into 2 round loaves. Place them in the prepared pans. Gently cut an inch-deep cross in the top of each.

Bake on the middle rack 30 to 35 minutes or until they are nicely browned and a wooden pick or cake tester inserted in the centers comes out clean. Remove the loaves from the pans and cool on wire racks before slicing. Wrapped in foil, the bread will freeze well.

Makes 2 loaves.

Old-Fashioned Oatmeal-Raisin Bread

This is a fabulous whole-grain breakfast bread, plain or toasted, with a little red currant jelly spread on top.

  2 tablespoons butter, cut into pieces
  2 tablespoons canola oil
 ½ cup packed dark brown sugar
1¾ cups uncooked regular or quick-cooking oatmeal
2½ cups hot water
  2 packages (5 teaspoons) active dry yeast
 ¾ teaspoon salt
 ¼ cup toasted wheat germ
  5 to 6 cups unbleached all-purpose flour
  1 cup raisins

Mix together the butter, oil, sugar, and oatmeal in the bowl of a heavy-duty electric mixer or other large bowl. Pour in the hot water and stir to blend. Let the mixture cool to lukewarm, then stir in the yeast. Let stand until the mixture bubbles, about 10 minutes.

Add the salt, wheat germ, and, gradually, enough flour to make a soft but manageable dough. Work in the raisins. Knead 5 minutes with an electric dough hook or 10 minutes by hand, until the dough is smooth and elastic.

Oil a large bowl and place dough in bowl, turning it to coat all sides. Cover and let dough rise in a warm place until doubled, about 1½ hours.

Spray 2 (9 × 5-inch) loaf pans with nonstick cooking spray. Punch the dough down, divide it in half, and form each half into a loaf shape. Place the loaves in the prepared pans and let them rise until doubled (almost to tops of pans), about 1½ hours.

Preheat the oven to 375F (190C). Bake the loaves on the middle rack about 45 minutes, or until they have risen and are browned and hollow-sounding when tapped on the bottom. Remove the bread from the pans, and allow to cool completely on a wire rack (see Notes opposite). Wrapped in foil, the bread will freeze well.

Makes 2 loaves.

NOTES

A loaf will lift quite easily out of the pan to test whether it sounds hollow when tapped on the bottom, but beware of the hot metal.

Do not slice the bread until it's cool. This is tough to do, since they'll smell scrumptious, but they'll keep much better if the moisture is retained inside.

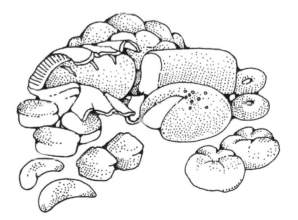

Whole-Grain "Power" Loaves

My idea of a "power" breakfast includes a toasted slice of this bread with a spoonful of ginger marmalade on top. If you're inspired to make the recipe but don't have on hand every last one of the grain ingredients, you can substitute one flour for another or flour for the flaxseed.

1 cup dried currants or raisins
1 package active dry yeast (2½ teaspoons)
2 cups warm water
2 cups unbleached all-purpose flour
2 cups whole-wheat flour
¾ cup whole-grain barley flour
1 cup whole-grain cornmeal
¼ cup milled flaxseed
¼ nonfat dry milk
¼ cup packed dark brown sugar
1½ teaspoons salt
¼ cup canola oil
2 tablespoons molasses
1 cup chopped hazelnuts or walnuts

Soak the currants in very hot water 5 minutes to plump them; drain.

Sprinkle the yeast on ½ cup of the warm water and let stand 5 minutes. Mix together the flours, cornmeal, flaxseed, dry milk, brown sugar, and salt in the large bowl of a heavy-duty electric mixer or other large bowl. Mix together yeast mixture, the remaining water, oil, and molasses in a small bowl. Beat the liquid ingredients into the dry ingredients until blended.

Knead 5 minutes with an electric dough hook or by hand 10 minutes, until the dough is smooth and elastic. Roll out the dough to a 1-inch-thick rectangle and scatter the currants and nuts over it. Roll up jelly-roll fashion, then keep folding the dough in half, and in half again, to distribute the currants and nuts throughout the dough. Expect a little resistance from this elastic dough.

Oil a large bowl and place dough in bowl, turning to coat all sides. Cover and let dough rise in a warm place until doubled, about 1½ to 2 hours.

Spray 2 (9 × 5-inch) loaf pans with nonstick cooking spray. Punch the dough down and form it into 2 loaves. Place the loaves in the prepared pans and let them rise until doubled (almost to tops of pans), about 1½ hours.

Preheat the oven to 350F (175C). Bake the loaves on the middle rack until they are brown on top and sound hollow when tapped on the bottom, 35 to 45 minutes. Remove from the pans and cool completely on wire racks before slicing.

Makes 2 loaves.

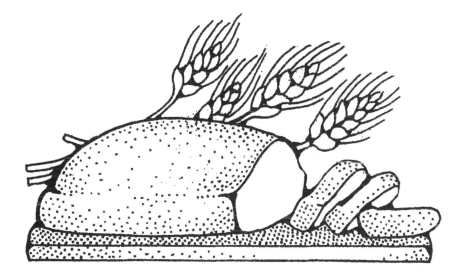

Pizza, the Healthy Way

Here's a pizza you can enjoy without guilt—low in fat and rich in the good nutrition of flax and vegetables. The instructions are long but not complicated, and the more often you make pizza at home, the easier it becomes. And it's a great Sunday night supper!

Pizza Dough
1 envelope active dry yeast (2½ teaspoons)
1 cup warm water
3 cups unbleached all-purpose flour
¼ cup milled flaxseed or wheat germ
½ teaspoon salt
2 tablespoons olive oil
  Cornmeal, for pan

Topping
2 cups thick tomato sauce, such as Baked Tomato Sauce (page 324), or from a jar
  Dried oregano
8 ounces part-skim shredded mozzarella cheese

Sprinkle the yeast on the warm water and let stand 5 minutes. Mix together the flour, flax, and salt in the bowl of a heavy-duty electric mixer or other large bowl. Stir in the oil until well blended. Stir in the yeast mixture to form a soft dough. If the dough does not form a ball, add 1 or 2 tablespoons more warm water as needed.

Knead the dough 5 minutes with a dough hook or 10 minutes by hand, until it's smooth and elastic. Oil a large bowl. Place the dough in bowl, turn to coat all sides, and cover with plastic wrap. Let rise until doubled, about 1 hour.

Punch down dough and divide it in half. Oil 2 (12-inch) pizza pans and dust them with cornmeal. Roll out the dough to fit the pans and place dough in pans. Cover and let rise again, 20 to 45 minutes, depending on whether you like a thin or thick pizza.

Preheat the oven to 425F (220C) or follow the instructions that came with your pizza pans: Different pans can require different temperatures. Position both racks in the bottom third of the oven.

Spread each crust with sauce to within 1 inch of the edge. Sprinkle with oregano to taste and the mozzarella cheese, dividing it between the two pizzas.

Arrange the pizzas on the two racks so that the top one covers as little as possible of the bottom one. Bake 10 minutes. Reverse the pizzas and continue baking about 8 minutes more, or until they are browned and crispy on the bottom and bubbling and golden on top. Remove from the pans and slice into 8 pieces per pizza.

Makes 16 slices; 8 servings.

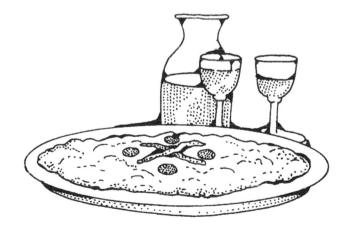

Bell Pepper, Olive, and Feta Focaccia

This focaccia has a savory Greek flavor.

 1 recipe Pizza Dough (page 184)
 1 red bell pepper, roasted, peeled (page 155), and cut into strips
 1 green bell pepper, roasted, peeled (page 155), and cut into strips
 1 tablespoon olive oil
 1 garlic clove, minced or pressed through a garlic press
 ¼ teaspoon salt
12 pitted kalamata olives, halved
 1 cup (about 3 oz.) loosely packed crumbled feta cheese
 1 tablespoon chopped fresh oregano or 1 teaspoon dried
    Freshly ground black pepper

Make the pizza dough as directed. While it is going through its first rise, mix the bell peppers with the oil, garlic, and salt, and let them stand at room temperature until needed.

Roll out the dough to fit 2 (10-inch-round) pizza pans. Cover and let rise until quite thick and breadlike, about 1 hour.

Preheat the oven to 425F (220C).

Use a brush to gently paint each focaccia with the reserved oil and garlic pieces. Arrange bell pepper strips on each round, alternating colors, like the spokes of a wheel. Divide the olive halves between the rounds. Sprinkle with feta cheese, dividing it between the rounds. Sprinkle them with the oregano. Season with pepper to taste.

Bake the focaccias on the bottom rack 18 minutes or until golden brown on the bottom and lightly colored on top. Remove from the pans and cut into 6 slices each.

Makes 12 slices; 6 servings.

Rosemary and Garlic Focaccia

Focaccia is an Italian flatbread, capable of infinite variety. This is one of the simplest versions, a wonderful accompaniment to soup. Rosemary and garlic are both rich in defensive phytochemicals. Use coarse kosher salt because the crystals will not melt during baking.

1 recipe Pizza Dough (page 184)
3 tablespoons olive oil
2 garlic cloves, minced or pressed through a garlic press
1 tablespoon chopped fresh rosemary or 1 teaspoon dried
   Kosher salt
   Freshly ground black pepper

Make the pizza dough as directed. While it is going through its first rise, mix the oil and garlic in a small dish and let them stand at room temperature.

Roll out the dough to fit 2 (10-inch-round) pizza pans. Cover and let rise until quite thick and breadlike, about 1 hour.

Preheat the oven to 425F (220C).

Use a brush to gently paint each focaccia with the garlic-flavored oil and garlic pieces. Sprinkle them with the rosemary. Season with salt and pepper to taste.

Bake the focaccias on the bottom rack 18 minutes, or until golden brown on the bottom and lightly colored on top. Remove from the pans and cut into 6 slices each.

Makes 12 slices; 6 servings.

Vegetables for a Vigorous Life

People who eat the most vegetables live longer . . . live healthier . . . and live smarter—that's the bottom line in not just one but many recent research studies. Scientists are not sure why this is so, but it appears that at least some of the answers may be found in the emerging field of phytochemicals. Along with these "vitamins of the future," some old favorites—antioxidant vitamins, B vitamins, and assorted minerals—have also been the subjects of studies providing new insights into the vegetable-health connection.

As for which vegetables carry what benefits, here are some of the winning groups. Vegetables rich in orange and red carotenoids (carrots, tomatoes) protect against many cancers. So do cruciferous vegetables (broccoli, cabbage). Soluble fiber (okra, onions) and flavonoids (artichokes, sweet potatoes) in some vegetables may reduce the risk of heart disease. Potassium-rich vegetables (asparagus, beans) help to avert strokes. Leafy green vegetables (kale, spinach) lessen the chance of blindness due to macular degeneration. From the B vitamin group, B_1 (corn, peas), B_6 (lentils, soybeans), and folate (beets, cauliflower) are important to perception, memory, judgment, and reasoning.

If you value "crunch," you'll want to buy fresh vegetables as often as possible, and locally grown are best. Exposure to air, heat, and light can lessen the vitamin content of "fresh" vegetables shipped across the country. Frozen vegetables are a good second choice, since they're processed before exposure reduces their vitamin value.

All fresh vegetables should be rinsed thoroughly under cool running water. Don't wash produce with detergent, however, since it may not rinse off completely. Outer leaves of headed vegetables, such as cabbage and iceberg lettuce, should be removed and discarded. Edible peels, which contain much of the vegetable's fiber and phytochemicals, should be scrubbed with a vegetable brush. Try to buy unwaxed vegetables, because wax can seal in traces of fungicides. Unfortunately, waxed vegetables should be peeled, even if they're ordinarily completely edible.

Your best chance to buy unwaxed vegetables, again, is to choose locally grown produce, which doesn't have to be shipped far and therefore doesn't need all that "protection." That will mean learning to value seasonal abundance. I find that following the growing cycles of vegetables can be a nice way of celebrating the seasons. Where I live, that would be a feast of asparagus in spring and a plenitude of squash in the fall.

Organic vegetables and fruits, while they cost more and are probably no more nutritious, are raised without chemical fertilizers, pesticides, fungicides, and herbicides. After harvesting, the produce isn't treated with wax or any artificial "enhancer." These are a lot of plusses. Do they taste better? You be the judge—try the oranges!

Some of the following recipes make vegetable dishes that could qualify as vegetarian entrees. Many others make nutritious, easy-to-prepare side dishes. Among these abundant plant foods, there is so much variety from which to choose, even the least enthusiastic vegetable eater should be able to enjoy something from every category.

Artichoke Hearts with Fennel

You can serve this as a vegetable side dish or as a sauce for Make-It-Easy Polenta (page 326) with freshly grated Parmesan cheese as an accompaniment.

  2 tablespoons olive oil
  1 large (about 1 lb.) fennel bulb, cored and cut into 1-inch chunks
  ¼ cup chopped shallots
  2 cups peeled, seeded, and chopped tomatoes
  4 strips lemon peel (with no white pith)
  ½ teaspoon salt
  ¼ teaspoon freshly ground black pepper
  1 (9-oz.) package frozen artichoke hearts, thawed to separate, and halved lengthwise
  1 tablespoon minced fresh basil, 2 teaspoons Basil Pesto (page 327), or ½ teaspoon dried basil

Heat the oil in a large skillet over medium-low heat and slowly sauté the fennel and shallots until lightly colored, 10 minutes. Add the tomatoes, lemon peel, salt, and pepper. Cover and simmer until the fennel is nearly tender, 10 minutes. If the tomatoes are not very juicy, you may need to add ¼ cup water. Add the artichoke hearts and simmer 5 minutes longer, or until everything is tender. Stir in the basil and cook 1 minute.

Makes 4 servings.

Asparagus with Fried Brown Rice

Brown rice offers a bonus of fiber and B vitamins. It takes a long time to cook, which is a good reason for making twice as much as you need. It will keep three to four days in the refrigerator. Leftovers make it easy to whip up another stir-fry.

1 pound fresh asparagus
2 tablespoons canola oil
4 scallions, sliced diagonally into 1-inch pieces
1 red bell pepper, seeded and cut into triangles
1 teaspoon minced fresh ginger
3 cups cooked, cooled brown rice
2 tablespoons soy sauce

Trim off the woody ends of the asparagus, and rinse the stalks well. Lay them in a large skillet with about ½ inch salted water. Bring to a boil, cover, and reduce heat. Cook until crisp-tender, 2 to 3 minutes, depending on the thickness of the stalks. Undercook slightly for this dish. Drain and rinse the stalks in cold water (in the skillet is the easiest way) until they are no longer warm. Drain again. Lay them on a cutting board and cut diagonally into 2-inch slices.

Heat the oil in a large skillet over medium-high heat. Stir-fry the scallions, bell pepper, and ginger until the vegetables are crisp-tender, about 3 minutes. Add the asparagus and rice. Stir-fry gently to heat through. Season with soy sauce and serve hot.

Makes 4 servings.

Greek-Style Green Beans

Fresh summer tomatoes combined with lots of onion give this dish a sweet piquancy.

1 tablespoon olive oil
1 large yellow onion, chopped
1 red bell pepper, seeded and diced
2 cups peeled, seeded, and chopped fresh tomatoes
1 pound green beans, cut diagonally into 2-inch lengths
1 tablespoon chopped fresh marjoram or ½ teaspoon dried oregano
½ teaspoon salt
   Freshly ground black pepper

Heat the oil in a large skillet over medium heat and sauté the onion and bell pepper until they begin to soften, about 5 minutes. Add the tomatoes and cook, stirring often, until the mixture reaches a sauce consistency, 8 to 10 minutes. Add the green beans, marjoram, and salt. Cover and simmer over low heat until the beans are quite tender, 8 to 10 minutes. Season with pepper to taste.

Makes 4 servings.

Swedish Green Beans with Dill-Mustard Sauce

Generally available in supermarkets all year, fresh dill is preferred in this simple dish.

  1 pound fresh green beans
  1 cup Chicken-Mushroom Stock (page 333) or canned broth
  1 tablespoon cornstarch
  1 teaspoon dry mustard
 ⅓ cup cold water
  2 tablespoons chopped fresh dill or 2 teaspoons dried
     White pepper

Trim the ends from the green beans. Slice them or not, as you wish. Cook the beans in a pot of boiling, salted water until crisp-tender, 5 to 7 minutes. Drain and rinse in cool water to stop the cooking.

Heat the stock to boiling in a large saucepan. Mix the cornstarch and dry mustard with the cold water until smooth. Add all at once to the boiling stock and cook, stirring constantly, until thickened. Reduce heat and add the dill and white pepper to taste. Simmer 1 to 2 minutes, then add the beans. Simmer 1 minute to combine flavors.

Makes 4 servings.

Chili Bean Dip

As an appetizer or a television-watching snack, this dip offers great nutrients instead of fat.

1 garlic clove, peeled and halved
1 (14- to 16-oz.) can pinto beans, drained and rinsed, or 2 cups cooked (page 328)
1 tablespoon chopped mild or hot chiles, either canned or fresh (see Note page 120 for handling hot chiles)
1 to 2 teaspoons chili powder, to taste
About 2 tablespoons fresh lime juice
Raw vegetables, crackers, or baked tortilla chips

With the motor running, drop the garlic down the feed tube of a processor to mince it. Add all the remaining ingredients and process to puree and blend. Stop the motor and scrape down the sides once or twice. Add enough lime juice to make a smooth spread.

Transfer dip to a bowl, cover, and refrigerate for several hours to combine flavors. Bring to room temperature before serving. Serve with vegetables, crackers, or baked tortilla chips.

Makes about 2 cups.

Kale with Black-eyed Peas

If you happen to have any leftover cooked sausage, slice and add it to this dish.

¾ pound kale, washed thoroughly, tough stems removed
     and chopped
 1 cup water
½ to 1 vegetable or chicken bouillon cube (see Note below)
 2 tablespoons olive oil
 2 garlic cloves, minced
 1 (14- to 16-oz.) can black-eyed peas, drained and rinsed, or 2 cups
     cooked (page 328)
¼ to ½ teaspoon hot red pepper flakes

Combine the kale, water, and bouillon cube in a large heavy pot. Cover and simmer until the kale is tender, 10 to 15 minutes. Drain, reserving the cooking water.

Heat the oil in a large skillet over medium heat and sauté the garlic until it's sizzling and fragrant but not brown, about 3 minutes. Add the kale and black-eyed peas, and season with pepper flakes to taste. Add about ¼ cup of the reserved cooking water to add moistness and toss to combine.

Makes 4 servings.

NOTE

Some bouillon cubes make 1 cup broth, and some make 2 cups. Read the package directions to determine how much bouillon you need for 1 cup broth.

Soybeans Caribbean

Nicely spicy! If you can't find soybeans at the supermarket, try a natural foods store—so much nutritional value is worth the effort!

2 (14- to 16-oz.) cans soybeans, drained and rinsed, or 3½ cups cooked (page 328)
1 (8-oz.) can juice-packed crushed pineapple, undrained
½ cup chili sauce
½ cup chopped scallions
2 tablespoons lime juice
1 tablespoon minced fresh ginger or 1 teaspoon ground ginger
1 teaspoon dry mustard

Preheat the oven to 375F (190C). Combine all the ingredients in a medium casserole dish. Bake until bubbling throughout, about 20 minutes. Serve hot.

Makes 4 servings.

Mediterranean Stir-Fry

Not all stir-fries are Asian.

3 cups broccoli flowerets with short, thin stems (about ½ inch wide, 2 inches long)
1 large red bell pepper, seeded and cut into triangles
2 garlic cloves, finely chopped
2 cups cooked, cooled brown rice
4 leaves fresh basil, slivered
¼ teaspoon salt
  Freshly ground black pepper
2 tablespoons freshly grated Romano cheese

Parboil the broccoli in boiling salted water 2 minutes. Drain.

Heat the oil in a large wok or skillet over high heat and stir-fry the bell pepper 1 minute. Add the garlic and cook 1 minute. Add the broccoli and stir-fry until the vegetables are crisp-tender, 2 to 3 minutes. Add the rice, basil, salt, and black pepper to taste. Heat through, tossing to blend the mixture. Sprinkle with cheese and serve.

Makes 4 servings.

Broccoli with Golden Garlic Crumbs and Pine Nuts

Broccoli "crowns" are sold in many supermarkets. They are the tops of the broccoli without the coarser stalks.

3 to 4 broccoli crowns (about 1 pound), cut into flowerets with short
   pieces of stalk attached
2 tablespoons olive oil
1 garlic clove, pressed through a garlic press
1 cup fresh bread crumbs (from 1 slice Italian bread)
½ cup pine nuts
   Salt and freshly ground black pepper

Cook the broccoli in a large pot of boiling salted water until crisp-tender, about 3 minutes. Drain.

Heat the oil in a large skillet over medium heat and stir in the garlic. Add the crumbs and stir-fry until they are golden, about 3 minutes. Add the pine nuts during the last minute.

If necessary, reheat the broccoli and spoon it into a flat serving dish with a lip. Season with salt and pepper to taste. Top with the crumb mixture and serve immediately.

Makes 4 servings.

Broccoli with Red Bell Pepper and Lemon

This simple dish is my favorite way to serve broccoli. The lemon is added last in order to preserve the bright green color of the broccoli.

1   bunch (about 1 lb.) broccoli
2   tablespoons olive oil
1   red bell pepper, seeded and cut into strips
1   garlic clove, minced
    Hot red pepper flakes
    Lemon wedges

Separate the broccoli into stalks with flowerets attached. Trim off any woody portion and peel the remainder of the stalks. Cut the stalks lengthwise to make them about ½ inch thick with flowerets still attached. Cook the broccoli in a large pot of boiling salted water until it is crisp-tender, about 3 minutes. Drain and refresh under cool water to stop the cooking action.

Heat the oil in a large skillet and stir-fry the bell pepper until it's crisp-tender, about 3 minutes. Add the garlic and cook 1 minute. Add the broccoli, and stir gently. Season with pepper flakes to taste and spoon the broccoli into a serving dish. Garnish with lemon wedges. Serve at room temperature.

Makes 4 servings.

Red Cabbage with Pears

A simple and tasty way to serve an important cruciferous vegetable.

1 very small head (about 1 lb.) red cabbage, thinly sliced
2 firm Bosc pears, peeled, cored, and thinly sliced
1 cup water
2 tablespoons cider vinegar or to taste
2 teaspoons sugar
½ teaspoon salt

Combine all the ingredients in a large saucepan. Bring to a simmer, cover, and cook 10 to 15 minutes, until the cabbage is tender but not mushy. Taste and correct seasoning; you may want more vinegar.

Makes 4 servings.

Carrots Vichy

A simple cooking method that imparts a mild, sweet flavor to winter carrots. In the folk wisdom of France, carrots were thought to be beneficial to the liver, and this dish was served often at Vichy, a French spa where the waters were also taken for hepatic conditions.

2 cups sliced carrots, about ½ inch thick
2 tablespoons butter
3 tablespoons water
1 teaspoon sugar
   Salt and freshly ground white pepper
1 tablespoon minced fresh flat-leaf parsley

Cook the carrots in boiling salted water until they are almost tender, about 5 minutes. Drain and rinse in cold water.

Melt the butter in a medium skillet over medium heat, and toss the carrots in it until they are well-coated. Add the water, sugar, salt, and pepper, and cook, stirring constantly, about 5 minutes, until the liquid has evaporated and the carrots are glazed. Sprinkle with parsley and serve hot.

Makes 4 servings.

Carrots Julienne with Lemon and Almonds

To cut rounded vegetables safely, first cut them (very carefully) in half lengthwise, then put the flat sides down on the cutting board for the rest of the slicing.

½ tablespoon butter
 4 large carrots, cut into julienne sticks
¼ cup water
    Dash of salt
½ teaspoon grated lemon peel
 2 tablespoons fresh lemon juice
 2 tablespoons slivered almonds, toasted (page 298)
    White pepper

Melt the butter in a medium saucepan over medium heat and stir-fry the carrots until they are coated and shining. Add the water and salt, and cook, stirring, until the carrots are crisp-tender, about 5 minutes after the water boils, adding more if necessary. Stir in the lemon peel and cook about 1 minute. Transfer to a warm serving dish. Stir in the lemon juice, almonds, and white pepper to taste.

Makes 4 servings.

Carrots and Green Beans with Fresh Herbs

A pretty and pleasing combination.

1 tablespoon butter
1 garlic clove, minced
1 pound fresh green beans, trimmed and cut diagonally into
    1-inch pieces
4 carrots, cut diagonally into ½-inch pieces
    About ¾ cup chicken broth
2 tablespoons fresh lemon juice
¼ teaspoon grated lemon peel
¼ teaspoon salt
⅛ teaspoon freshly ground black pepper
1 tablespoon chopped fresh chives
1 tablespoon chopped fresh marjoram
1 tablespoon chopped fresh parsley

Heat the butter in a large skillet over medium heat and sauté the garlic until softened but not brown, 3 minutes. Add the vegetables and broth, cover, and simmer until the vegetables are tender, about 10 minutes, adding more broth, if needed.

Blend the lemon juice and peel into the vegetables, distributing the peel well throughout. Season with salt and pepper. Toss with the herbs and serve.

Makes 6 servings.

Curried Cauliflower Mimosa

To hard-cook eggs without overcooking them and turning the whites green, put them in a saucepan with cold water to cover. Bring to a slow boil and cook 1 minute. Cover the pan and remove it from the heat. Let the eggs stand in the hot water 20 minutes. Then drain, crack the shells, and rinse in cool water.

- 1 large head cauliflower
- 1 tablespoon white vinegar
- ⅓ cup nonfat dry milk
- 3 tablespoons instant flour, such as Wondra
- 1 to 2 teaspoons curry powder or to taste
- ½ teaspoon salt
- 1½ cups low-fat milk
- ¼ teaspoon white pepper
- 1 tablespoon chopped fresh cilantro
- 2 large hard-cooked eggs, coarsely chopped
  Cilantro sprigs, for garnish (optional)

Trim off the leaves and core and separate the cauliflower into flowerets. Cut any extra-large flowerets in half. Cook the cauliflower with the white vinegar in a large pot of boiling salted water until crisp-tender, about 3 minutes. Drain.

Mix together the dry milk, flour, curry powder, and salt, then whisk the dry ingredients into the liquid milk in a saucepan. Bring the mixture to a boil over medium-high heat, stirring constantly, until it's bubbling and thickened. Reduce heat to very low, and simmer 3 minutes, stirring often. Stir in the white pepper, chopped cilantro, and chopped eggs.

Arrange the cauliflower in a serving dish and pour the curry sauce over it. Garnish with cilantro sprigs, if desired.

Makes 6 servings.

Savory Cauliflower with Anchovies and Garlic

If you don't love anchovies, you can make this dish without them. Just double up on the sun-dried tomatoes.

1 large head cauliflower
1 tablespoon white vinegar
2 tablespoons olive oil
4 anchovies, chopped
1 garlic clove, minced
1 tablespoon capers, drained
4 oil-packed sun-dried tomatoes, drained and slivered
  Freshly ground black pepper
2 tablespoons chopped fresh flat-leaf parsley

Trim off the leaves and core and separate the cauliflower into flowerets. Cut any extra-large flowerets in half. Cook the cauliflower with the white vinegar in a large pot of boiling salted water until crisp-tender, about 3 minutes. Drain.

Warm the oil in a large skillet over low heat and warm the anchovies in it until they begin to dissolve, chopping them with the side of a spoon. Add the garlic and cook 1 minute. Add the cauliflower, capers, tomatoes, and pepper to taste, and toss to blend. Cook over low heat 1 to 2 minutes, stirring often. Stir in the parsley.

Serve at room temperature.

Makes 4 servings.

Sesame Cauliflower

Sesame is a rich source of vitamin E and selenium.

1 tablespoon soy sauce
1 tablespoon sesame seeds, crushed slightly in a mortar with a pestle
1 teaspoon sesame oil
½ teaspoon salt
2 tablespoons canola oil
1 bunch scallions, white parts only, sliced into 1-inch pieces
1 small head cauliflower, trimmed and separated into flowerets
   about 1 inch wide

Combine the soy sauce, sesame seeds, sesame oil, and salt in a cup.
Heat the canola oil in a large skillet over medium heat and sauté the scallions 1 minute. Add the cauliflower and stir-fry 3 minutes. Add the soy
mixture, tossing with the vegetables to coat them evenly. Cook over very
low heat, stirring often, until the cauliflower is crisp-tender, about 5
minutes, adding 1 tablespoon water to the pan, if necessary.
Makes 4 servings.

Creamy Corn and Bell Pepper Pudding

This makes a lovely side dish with chicken, or a luncheon dish all on its own.

1 tablespoon olive oil
1 tablespoon butter
1 small green bell pepper, seeded and diced
1 small yellow onion, diced
2 egg whites
   Pinch of cream of tartar
1⅓ cups low-fat milk
2 egg yolks
3 tablespoons all-purpose flour
¼ teaspoon salt
⅛ teaspoon cayenne pepper
2 cups fresh or frozen whole-kernel corn, cooked

Preheat the oven to 325F (165C). Butter a 2-quart casserole dish.

Heat the olive oil and butter in a small skillet over medium heat and sauté the bell pepper and onion until tender, 5 minutes.

Beat the egg whites until foamy. Add the cream of tartar and continue beating until the whites are stiff but not dry.

Beat together the milk, egg yolks, flour, salt, and cayenne. Stir in the corn and sautéed vegetables. Fold in the beaten egg whites. Pour the mixture into the prepared casserole dish, and set it in a larger pan. Pour hot water into the outside pan. Bake the pudding until just set, about 45 minutes. Serve immediately.

Makes 4 servings.

Eggplant and Roasted Garlic Caviar

Easily roasted together, eggplant and garlic develop a deeply delicious flavor. Pricking the eggplant before baking prevents the pressure of trapped steam from exploding it in your oven.

1 large eggplant
1 large garlic bulb
2 tablespoons olive oil
2 tablespoons fresh lemon juice
½ teaspoon salt
¼ teaspoon freshly ground black pepper
¼ cup minced fresh flat-leaf parsley
1 tablespoon minced fresh marjoram or 1 teaspoon dried oregano
   Crudités and/or pita bread

Preheat the oven to 375F (190C). Prick the eggplant in several places with a fork and place it on a baking sheet. Cut the top off the garlic bulb, wrap the bulb in foil, and place it on the same baking sheet. Bake the vegetables 35 to 40 minutes, turning eggplant once; the eggplant may be tender before the garlic, in which case, remove it from the oven. For a rich flavor it's important that the eggplant be soft and yield a little when pressed with the back of a cooking spoon. The garlic should be squeezable.

Cool the vegetables. Peel the eggplant and cut up the flesh. Squeeze each garlic clove out of its skin. Puree the eggplant and garlic in a food processor. Add the oil, lemon juice, salt, and pepper and process until smooth. Transfer the puree to a bowl and stir in the herbs. Serve with crudités or pita bread or both.

Makes 2 cups.

Eggplant Steaks with Mushrooms

This dish makes a substantial vegetarian entree.

1 very large (1½-lb.) eggplant
  About 3 tablespoons olive oil
1 garlic clove, pressed through a garlic press
6 large brown mushrooms, cleaned and sliced
  Salt and freshly ground black pepper
6 tablespoons Italian Marinara Sauce (page 321) or from a jar
6 teaspoons seasoned bread crumbs
6 teaspoons freshly grated Parmesan cheese

Trim off the ends and peel the eggplant. Slice it lengthwise into 6 even slices. Salt the slices and allow them to drain in a colander about 30 minutes.

Meanwhile, combine the olive oil and garlic and let stand.

Preheat the broiler. Rinse and press the eggplant slices to squeeze out moisture. Pat them dry between layers of paper towels. Brush them on both sides with the garlic oil, and arrange them in a single layer on a baking sheet. Broil them on the top rack until slightly browned and tender, 4 to 5 minutes per side. Leave the eggplant on the baking sheet and set aside.

Turn off broiler. Set oven temperature at 400F (205C).

Heat remaining garlic oil in a medium nonstick skillet over high heat and sauté the mushrooms, stirring often, until they begin to brown, adding more olive oil, if needed. Season with salt and pepper to taste; set aside.

Spread each eggplant slice with 1 tablespoon of sauce, then sprinkle with 1 teaspoon of crumbs and 1 teaspoon of cheese. Bake until the cheese is slightly browned, about 5 minutes. Top each slice with mushrooms.

Makes 3 servings.

Lighter Eggplant Parmesan

Leftovers make a great sandwich filling.

  1 large (1- to 1¼-lbs.) eggplant
  1 garlic clove, crushed
  2 tablespoons olive oil
1½ cups of the Italian tomato sauces (pages 320–21) or
       any sauce from a jar
  ¼ cup freshly grated Parmesan cheese

Peel, slice, and salt the eggplant. Allow the slices to drain in a colander about 30 minutes.

Meanwhile, combine the garlic and oil and let stand.

Preheat the oven to 450F (230C). Rinse and press dry the eggplant slices. Discard garlic and brush the oil on both sides of the eggplant slices. Arrange them in a single layer on a baking sheet. Bake on the top rack of the oven 8 minutes, or until tender and lightly colored.

Reduce oven temperature to 375F (190C). Spread about ¼ of the sauce in a 9 × 9-inch baking dish. Add a layer of ⅓ of the eggplant. Top with ¼ of the sauce and 1 tablespoon cheese. Repeat with the remaining ingredients, ending with sauce and 2 tablespoons cheese. Bake, uncovered, 45 minutes or until the eggplant is very tender and the casserole is bubbly.

Serve warm or at room temperature.

Makes 4 servings.

Braised Fennel Parmesan

Like other members of the feathery-leafed umbelliferae *family, fennel contains cancer-fighting phytochemicals.*

    2 tablespoons olive oil
    2 fennel bulbs, quartered lengthwise and cored
    1 large shallot, chopped
    1 teaspoon fresh chopped oregano or marjoram
      Salt and freshly ground black pepper
 1½ cups chicken or vegetable broth
  ½ cup freshly grated Parmesan cheese

Heat the oil in a large skillet over medium heat and fry the fennel until it's lightly browned on both sides. Add the shallot and cook 1 minute. Sprinkle with oregano and season with salt and pepper to taste. Add the broth to the pan, cover, and simmer until the fennel is very tender, about 15 minutes.

Preheat the broiler. Transfer the fennel to a flameproof baking dish and sprinkle with the cheese. Broil until the cheese is melted, 3 to 5 minutes.

Makes 4 servings.

Broccoli Rabe and Chick-Peas

Delicious as a side dish or served over Orzo and Rice Pilaf (page 146) as a vegetable entree.

1   bunch (¾ lb.) broccoli rabe (rapini), well-washed and tough
   ends trimmed
1   cup Vegetable Stock (page 331), Chicken-Mushroom Stock
   (page 333), or canned broth
2   tablespoons olive oil
1   medium yellow onion, chopped
½   cup Italian Marinara Sauce (page 321) or from a jar
1   (14- to 16-oz.) can chick-peas, drained and rinsed, or 2 cups
   cooked (page 328)
¼   teaspoon hot red pepper flakes

Hold the broccoli rabe together in a bunch and cut it crosswise into quarters. Put it into a pot with the stock and bring to a simmer. Cook, covered, until the rabe is tender, 10 minutes.

Meanwhile, heat the oil in a large skillet and sauté the onion over medium heat until it's soft, 5 minutes. Add the tomato sauce and chick-peas and simmer 5 minutes.

Using a slotted spoon, transfer the rabe to the chick-pea mixture. Add ¼ cup of the rabe stock to the skillet. Stir in pepper flakes. Simmer 2 to 3 minutes over very low heat to blend flavors.

Makes 4 servings.

Braised Chard with Brown Rice

Other leafy greens can be substituted for the chard in this recipe. Make the rice in advance, since it takes much longer to cook. Keep it warm, or reheat if cold.

1 large bunch (1¼ lbs.) fresh chard, well-washed
2 tablespoons olive oil
2 garlic cloves, minced
  Salt and freshly ground black pepper
2½ cups hot cooked brown rice
  Lemon wedges (optional)

Reassemble the chard into a bunch and chop it. Slice the stems cross-wise into pieces about 1 inch wide and cut the leaves into pieces about 2 inches wide.

Heat the oil in a large pot and sauté the garlic over medium heat until it's sizzling and fragrant. Add the chard and stir-fry until wilted, about 5 minutes. If the leaves are not still wet from washing, add 2 to 3 table-spoons water. Cover the pan and simmer over low heat 10 minutes or until tender. Season with salt and pepper.

Make a ring of the rice in a large serving dish and spoon the chard into the center. If you wish, pass lemon wedges at the table.

Makes 4 servings.

Buttered Turnip Greens and Corn with Hazelnuts

Chopped hazelnuts used to be a chore to prepare, but now that they're sold shelled in bags at the supermarket, they're much easier to use as an enrichment of flavor, crunch, and boron, a bone mineral.

1   bunch (about 1 lb.) turnip greens, well-washed and chopped
1   cup Vegetable Stock (page 331), Chicken-Mushroom Stock (page 333), or canned broth
2   tablespoons butter
2   cups fresh or frozen whole-kernel corn
⅓   cup chopped hazelnuts
1   tablespoon chopped fresh chives

Put the greens, stock, and butter into a large saucepan over medium heat. Bring to a simmer, cover, and cook until the greens are nearly tender, 10 to 15 minutes. Taste is the best test; mature greens take longer. Add the corn and cook 5 minutes longer. Stir in the hazelnuts and chives before serving.

Makes 4 servings.

Spinach with Ripe Olives on Whole-Wheat Couscous

When you add olives to a dish, you probably won't need any additional salt.

10 ounces fresh spinach
 1 tablespoon olive oil
 1 garlic clove, minced
12 Greek or French black olives, pitted and halved
    Freshly ground black pepper
 2 cups Chicken-Mushroom Stock (page 333) or canned broth
 1 cup uncooked whole-wheat couscous (see Note below)

Wash the spinach well, remove the tough stems, and chop it coarsely. Heat the oil in a large skillet over medium heat and sauté the garlic until it sizzles. Add the spinach, still wet from its washing, and cover. Cook over low heat until wilted, 2 to 3 minutes, stirring often. Stir in the olives. Season with pepper to taste.

Meanwhile, bring the stock to a boil in the top of a double boiler over medium heat. Gradually add the couscous, and cook, stirring, until the mixture returns to a boil. Place top of double boiler over 1 inch of simmering water, cover, and cook 15 minutes. Uncover and fluff well. Spoon the couscous onto a medium serving platter and break up any remaining clumps. Top with the spinach.

Makes 4 servings.

NOTE

If you substitute refined white couscous, follow the package directions. White couscous only needs to be combined with the boiling stock and allowed to stand until all the liquid is absorbed. Whole-wheat couscous, on the other hand, should be cooked as described in the recipe.

Creamed Spinach, Spanish Style

"Creamed" dishes can be made a lot lighter by using low-fat milk instead of cream in the sauce.

2 (10-oz.) packages fresh spinach, well-washed and tough stems removed, or 2 (10-oz.) packages frozen leaf spinach
½ cup chicken broth or water
1 tablespoon olive oil
2 shallots, chopped
2 tablespoons butter
3 tablespoons all-purpose flour
1 cup hot low-fat or whole milk
¼ teaspoon salt
¼ teaspoon white pepper
⅛ teaspoon cayenne pepper
⅛ teaspoon ground nutmeg
Juice of ½ large lime
1 cup fresh bread crumbs (from 1 slice Italian bread)

Put the fresh spinach and broth in a large pot and bring to a boil. Cover and simmer until the spinach is wilted, about 5 minutes. Drain the spinach, reserving cooking liquid. If using frozen spinach, follow the package directions.

Heat the oil in a medium saucepan over medium heat and sauté the shallots, stirring often, until sizzling and fragrant, about 3 minutes. Add the butter, and when it has melted, stir in the flour. Cook over very low heat, stirring constantly, 2 to 3 minutes. Add the hot milk, all at once, increase heat to medium-high, and cook, stirring constantly, until the mixture is thick and beginning to bubble. (It will be quite thick.) Whisk in the salt, white pepper, cayenne, nutmeg, lime juice, and ¼ cup of the reserved cooking liquid. Simmer over very low heat 3 minutes, stirring often.

Position the top oven rack 6 inches below the heat source and preheat the broiler. Chop the spinach and put it into a flameproof gratin dish. Pour the sauce over the spinach and sprinkle with the crumbs. Broil until the mixture bubbles and the crumbs are golden, about 5 minutes.

Makes 6 servings.

Roasted Whole Onions, Sicilian Style

A simple but unusual side dish. Onions ward off infections from bacteria and viruses, and they're rich in soluble fiber for the heart.

6   yellow onions, all about the same size
1   tablespoon olive oil
1   sprig of fresh thyme
1   sprig of fresh sage
    Lemon wedges
    Salt and freshly ground pepper

Preheat the oven to 350F (175C).

Rinse the onions. Cut a ¼-inch-thick slice off each stem end; leave the peels and root ends intact. Place the onions, cut sides up, in a baking pan that will hold them upright and drizzle them with the oil. Arrange the herb sprigs on top of the onions.

Cut a piece of foil large enough to cover onions and cut 3 slits in it. Cover the onions loosely with the foil. Bake until the onions are quite tender, 1 to 1½ hours. Serve hot, cold, or at room temperature, accompanied by lemon wedges, salt, and pepper.

Makes 6 servings.

VARIATION

Roasted Onion Soup

For each leftover roasted onion, allow 1 cup beef broth and ½ tablespoon chopped fresh parsley. Peel and chop the onions. Combine the onions, broth, and parsley in a saucepan and simmer 3 minutes.

Meanwhile, make croutons: Toast 1 slice of Italian white bread for each serving. Rub it with a cut clove of garlic and sprinkle with grated Parmesan cheese. If you wish, you can put the croutons under a preheated broiler 1 minute to melt the cheese. Float a crouton on each serving of soup.

Leeks Gratin

An attractive side dish that's a real immunity booster.

8 leeks, white and light green parts only
1 cup chicken broth
3 tablespoons nonfat dry milk
3 tablespoons instant flour, such as Wondra
½ teaspoon salt
⅛ to ¼ teaspoon white pepper
1 cup low-fat or whole milk
1 tablespoon butter
½ cup slivered Gruyère cheese or 3 tablespoons freshly grated
   Parmesan cheese
2 tablespoons plain or seasoned dry bread crumbs

Slice the leeks in half lengthwise and carefully rinse between the rings to remove any sand without separating them. Combine the leeks and broth in a skillet, cover, and simmer until tender, about 15 minutes. Drain, reserving liquid. Lay the leeks in a gratin dish that will hold them in a single layer.

Preheat the oven to 375F (190C).

Whisk the dry milk, flour, salt, and white pepper into the liquid milk. Pour it into the same skillet and cook over medium-high heat, stirring constantly, until bubbling. It will be quite thick. Whisk in ¼ cup or more of the reserved cooking liquid from the leeks to make a smooth pourable sauce. Simmer over very low heat 3 minutes, stirring often. Swirl in the butter and cheese, and remove from the heat.

Pour the sauce over the leeks. Top with the crumbs. Bake 20 minutes or until lightly browned on top and bubbling throughout.

Makes 4 servings.

Peppers and Onions with Basil

Rich in vitamin C, this is a flavorful side dish to serve with any plain meat—burgers, chicken, or fish—and if differently colored bell peppers are used, it's decorative as well. Use fresh basil if available.

- 2 tablespoons olive oil
- 1 large yellow onion, peeled and sliced into half-rounds
- 1 garlic clove, finely diced
- 4 bell peppers, preferably a combination of colors (green, yellow, red), seeded and cut into chunks
- 6 to 8 leaves of fresh basil, slivered, or ½ teaspoon dried
    Salt and freshly ground black pepper

Heat the oil in a 12-inch skillet over medium heat and sauté the onion until soft, 5 minutes. Add the garlic and bell peppers, and sauté, stirring often and distributing the garlic evenly throughout, until the bell peppers are tender, 5 to 7 minutes more. Remove from the heat. Stir in the basil. Season with salt and pepper to taste.

Makes 4 servings.

VARIATIONS

Peppers with Walnuts

Prepare as above, adding 1/2 cup unsalted walnut halves or pieces with the basil. Use as a side dish or as a vegetarian sandwich filling in a pita pocket.

Peppers with Cherry Tomatoes

Prepare the bell peppers as in the original recipe. Gently stir 8 small cherry tomatoes, halved, into the bell peppers after they have cooked about 4 minutes.

As a side dish, transfer the hot vegetables to a serving dish and top with 1 cup shredded mozzarella cheese. Or for a quick pasta dish, stir the vegetables and mozzarella cheese into 8 ounces cooked medium pasta shells.

Scalloped Potatoes, Leeks, and Greens

Allicin foods like leeks lower LDL cholesterol and act as blood thinners, guarding against strokes. Niacin in potatoes and vitamin E in dark leafy greens make this an all-round heart-healthy dish.

1 tablespoon olive oil
2 large leeks, white and light green parts, chopped
2 cups Vegetable Stock (page 331), Chicken-Mushroom Stock (page 333), canned broth, or prepared bouillon
½ teaspoon salt
⅛ teaspoon freshly ground pepper
¼ teaspoon dried thyme
1 pound russet potatoes, cut into ¼-inch-thick slices
¾ pound mustard or turnip greens, tough stems removed, well-rinsed, and chopped

Preheat the oven to 375F (190C).

Heat the oil in a large pot over medium heat and sauté the leeks until they are softened and lightly colored, 5 to 8 minutes. Add the stock, salt, pepper, thyme, and potatoes. Cover and simmer 3 minutes (the potatoes should be only partly cooked).

With a slotted spoon, transfer the potatoes and leeks to a 2½-quart casserole dish. Add the greens to the pot and bring to a boil. As soon as the greens wilt, about 1 minute, remove them with a slotted spoon, and stir them gently into the potatoes. Pour in enough stock to come to within ½ inch of the top layer of vegetables.

Bake the casserole, uncovered, until the potatoes are very tender, 35 to 40 minutes.

Makes 4 servings.

Roasted Potatoes and Carrots

A crowd-pleasing dish that's easy to double or triple by using more than one pan.

3 large carrots, halved lengthwise and crosswise
4 large baking potatoes, peeled and quartered lengthwise
3 tablespoons olive oil
1 tablespoon chopped fresh marjoram or ½ teaspoon dried oregano
1 teaspoon fresh chopped rosemary or ¼ teaspoon dried
   Salt and freshly ground pepper

Preheat the oven to 400F (205C).

Parboil the carrots in boiling salted water 3 minutes. Drain well and blot dry with paper towels.

Combine the carrots and remaining ingredients in a large roasting pan, and toss to coat the vegetables with oil and seasonings. Arrange them in a single layer and bake, uncovered, in the top third of the oven until the vegetables are quite tender, 35 to 45 minutes, turning once; loosen carefully with a spatula to keep potato crusts intact.

Makes 4 to 6 servings.

Pan Potatoes with Rosemary and Chives

A flavorsome brunch or light supper dish that's sure to garner rave reviews. Covering the pan partially steams the potatoes so that they cook more quickly and thus require very little oil.

  2 tablespoons olive oil
  6 russet potatoes, peeled and thinly sliced
     Salt and freshly ground pepper
  2 teaspoons chopped fresh rosemary
  ¼ cup chopped fresh chives

Heat the oil in a 10-inch nonstick skillet over medium-low heat and layer in about half the potatoes. Salt and pepper them to taste, and sprinkle them with half the rosemary and chives. Repeat with the remaining potatoes, rosemary, and chives. Cover and fry potatoes, occasionally lifting the browned potatoes up and moving the unbrowned potatoes to the bottom of the skillet. Cook until tender, about 15 minutes.
Makes 4 servings.

VARIATION

Pan Potatoes with Onions

Follow the preceding recipe, omitting the chives and layering in 1 large yellow onion, sliced and separated into rings.

Sweet Potatoes with Cranberries

A colorful combination. Fresh cranberries have a short season, but you can buy several bags and freeze them to extend it.

1 cup fresh cranberries, picked over and rinsed
¾ cup orange juice
¼ cup sugar
2 pounds sweet potatoes, peeled and cut into 1-inch chunks

Combine the cranberries, orange juice, and sugar in a large heavy saucepan. Bring to a boil over medium heat, stirring to dissolve the sugar. Simmer, uncovered, stirring often, until the berries have popped, about 10 minutes.

Separately, steam the potatoes over boiling water until just tender, 10 to 12 minutes. Stir the potatoes into the cranberries and simmer them together 2 to 3 minutes.

Makes 4 servings.

Sweet Potatoes and Leeks Moroccan

A substantial dish rich in foods that build immunity.

  2 tablespoons olive oil
  3 large leeks, white and light green parts, rinsed and chopped
  1 slice fresh ginger, minced
  2 garlic cloves, minced
  1 cup peeled, seeded, chopped fresh tomatoes, or chopped canned
     tomatoes, undrained
½ cup chicken broth
  4 medium (about 2 lbs.) sweet potatoes, peeled and cut into
     1-inch chunks
½ teaspoon ground cumin
½ teaspoon ground coriander
¼ teaspoon salt
¼ teaspoon ground cinnamon
¼ teaspoon hot pepper sauce or to taste
     Hot cooked couscous (see Note, page 216)

Heat the oil in a Dutch oven over low heat and cook the leeks and ginger 5 to 8 minutes, until lightly colored. Add the garlic and sauté 1 minute. Add the tomatoes, broth, sweet potatoes, cumin, coriander, salt, cinnamon, and hot pepper sauce. Simmer, covered, until the vegetables are very tender, about 15 minutes, stirring occasionally. If the stew seems too dry, add a bit more broth.

Taste and correct seasoning; you may want more hot pepper sauce. Serve with couscous.

Makes 4 servings.

Sweet Potato and Apple Casserole

A make-now, cook-later dish that's perfect for winter holiday menus.

1 tablespoon canola oil
½ cup chopped onion
2 medium sweet potatoes, peeled and diced
1 cooking apple, such as Rome or Granny Smith, peeled and diced
½ cup chicken broth
¼ teaspoon dried rosemary
⅛ teaspoon dried thyme
¼ teaspoon salt
1 cup herb stuffing mix
Freshly ground nutmeg or allspice

Heat the oil in a medium saucepan over medium heat and sauté the onion until lightly colored, 3 to 4 minutes. Add the potatoes, apple, broth, herbs, and salt, and bring the mixture to a boil. Cover and simmer until the potatoes are just tender, 5 to 8 minutes. Transfer the mixture with the juices to a 2-quart gratin or casserole dish. (If making ahead, cover and refrigerate overnight.)

When ready to finish the dish, preheat the oven to 350F (175C). Sprinkle the top of the casserole with the stuffing mix, pressing it down into the moist potatoes, and add a few dashes of nutmeg or allspice. Bake until golden on top, 20 to 30 minutes, depending on whether you've refrigerated the dish between preparation and baking.

Makes 4 servings.

Gingery Pumpkin Casserole

Another delicious low-fat holiday dish that can be prepared in advance. Ginger offers relief to arthritis suffers because it inhibits prostaglandins, just as many anti-inflammatory drugs do.

A pumpkin shell is tough, so it's necessary to be extra careful with the knife in preparing it.

1 (2½- to 3-lb.) "sugar" pumpkin or butternut squash
½ cup walnut halves or pieces
2 tablespoons brown sugar
1 teaspoon ground ginger
½ teaspoon ground cinnamon
¼ teaspoon ground nutmeg
¼ teaspoon salt
2 tablespoons chopped crystallized ginger

Cut the pumpkin in half. Clean out the seeds and strings. Discard the stem. Cut the pumpkin into wedges. Steam the wedges over boiling water until the flesh is tender, 15 to 20 minutes. Let cool until they can be handled. Peel off the skin.

Put the walnuts into a saucepan with water to cover and bring to a boil. Drain and rinse the walnuts; set aside.

Puree the pumpkin in a food processor. Add the sugar, spices, and salt; pulse to blend. Alternatively, mash the pumpkin with a potato masher. Spoon the pumpkin mixture into a casserole dish and stir in the crystallized ginger. Scatter the walnuts over the top.

When ready to cook, preheat the oven to 350F (175C). Bake 20 to 25 minutes (30 to 35 if the dish has been refrigerated).

Makes 6 servings.

Pumpkin with Onions and Sage

Fresh sage is especially delicious in this simple dish, which can be adapted to any winter squash.

1 tablespoon olive oil
1 tablespoon unsalted butter
1 large yellow onion, chopped
1 celery stalk, chopped
1 cup Chicken-Mushroom Stock (page 333), Vegetable Stock (page 331), or canned broth
1½ pounds peeled, diced pumpkin or butternut squash
1 tablespoon fresh chopped sage leaves or ½ teaspoon dried leaves (not ground)
  Salt and freshly ground black pepper

Heat the oil and butter in a 10-inch skillet over medium heat and fry the onion and celery, stirring often, until they are golden, 5 to 7 minutes. Add the stock and pumpkin, cover, and cook until the pumpkin is tender, about 10 minutes. Stir in the sage. Season with salt and pepper to taste.

Makes 4 servings.

Gratin of Butternut Squash, Tomatoes, and Olives

Combining the carotenoids of orange and red vegetables, this dish is simple yet an interesting change from sweet squash dishes.

  1 large (2- to 2½-lb.) butternut squash, seeded, peeled, and
    cut into 1-inch chunks
½ cup ripe black olives, halved
  2 tablespoons olive oil
  1 garlic clove, minced
1½ cups peeled, seeded, chopped fresh or canned tomatoes
  2 tablespoons cornstarch
¼ teaspoon salt
⅛ teaspoon freshly ground black pepper
  1 cup vegetable broth
  1 tablespoon chopped fresh basil or 1 teaspoon dried
  1 cup fresh bread crumbs (from 1 slice crustless Italian bread)

Preheat the oven to 375F (190C). Oil a 13 × 9-inch gratin pan or a glass or ceramic baking dish.

Steam the squash chunks until nearly tender, 5 to 7 minutes. Put the squash into prepared pan. Scatter the olives on top; set aside.

Heat 1 tablespoon of the oil in a saucepan over medium heat and sauté the garlic until softened but not brown, 3 minutes. Add the tomatoes and cook 3 minutes. Whisk the cornstarch, salt, and pepper into the cold broth until well blended, and add cornstarch mixture to the tomatoes. Cook on medium-high heat, stirring constantly, until thick and bubbling. Reduce heat and simmer 2 minutes, stirring often. Remove pan from the heat and stir in the basil. Pour the sauce over the squash.

Sprinkle the bread crumbs over the sauce, and drizzle with the remaining 1 tablespoon of oil. Bake in the top third of the oven until golden brown and crusty, 20 to 30 minutes.

Makes 6 servings.

Roasted Butternut Squash and Yellow Potatoes

Yellow potatoes have a lovely mellow flavor that blends beautifully with squash.

  3 tablespoons olive oil
  2 garlic cloves, crushed
  1 pound butternut squash, peeled and cut into 1-inch cubes
  1 pound yellow potatoes, such as Yukon Gold, peeled and cut into 1-inch cubes
  ¼ teaspoon dried rosemary
  ¼ teaspoon dried oregano
     Salt and freshly ground black pepper

Preheat the oven to 375F (190C).

Combine the oil and garlic in a large roasting pan that will hold the vegetables in one layer. Add the squash and potatoes and stir to coat all sides. Season them with the herbs and salt and pepper to taste.

Bake in the top third of the oven until tender, 40 to 45 minutes, carefully turning vegetables once halfway through the cooking time. Remove and discard the garlic before serving.

Makes 4 servings.

Acorn Squash with Spinach and Feta

The neat shape of acorn squash seems to ask to be stuffed with a savory filling like this one.

 2 medium acorn squash
    Ground allspice
 2 cups cooked spinach, drained and liquid reserved
 1 cup herb stuffing mix
 1 teaspoon dried dill weed
 ½ cup crumbled feta cheese
    Salt and freshly ground black pepper

Preheat the oven to 400F (205C).

Cut the squash in half and clean out the seeds. Put the halves in a baking dish that will hold them upright, cut sides up. Sprinkle them with allspice. Add ½ inch of water to the pan. Bake the squash in the middle of the oven until tender, about 45 minutes.

Mix together all the remaining ingredients, with salt and pepper to taste. If necessary, add a little of the reserved spinach cooking liquid to moisten the stuffing so that it holds together. Divide the stuffing among the squash. At this point, they can be refrigerated for later baking, if desired.

Bake until heated through and golden on top, 20 to 25 minutes, 30 minutes if they have been refrigerated.

Makes 4 servings.

Brussels Sprouts with Horseradish Cream

Two assertive flavors (both cruciferous vegetables) make a complementary match.

1   pound fresh brussels sprouts, trimmed, or 1 (1-lb.) bag frozen
    brussels sprouts
1   tablespoon canola oil
1   medium yellow onion, chopped
1   to 2 tablespoons grated horseradish or to taste
½   cup nonfat plain yogurt, at room temperature

Cut a small cross in the stem of each sprout. Cook the sprouts in a large pot of boiling salted water until they are tender, about 8 minutes. If using frozen sprouts, cook them according to package directions. Drain the sprouts.

Heat the oil in a 10-inch nonstick skillet over medium heat and sauté the onion until soft, 5 minutes. Add the sprouts, and warm them with the onion to combine flavors.

Mix the horseradish with the yogurt. Toss the horseradish mixture with the warm sprouts and serve.

Makes 4 servings.

Brussels Sprouts Gratin with Rice

With its richness of cheese and milk, this dish could be considered a vegetable entree.

```
 1 pound fresh brussels sprouts, trimmed
 1 tablespoon butter
 2 tablespoons canola oil
¼ cup chopped shallots
 3 tablespoons unbleached all-purpose flour
1½ cups whole or low-fat milk, heated
 1 cup (4 oz.) shredded sharp Cheddar cheese
¼ teaspoon white pepper
 2 cups cooked brown rice
¼ cup plain bread or cracker crumbs
```

Preheat the oven to 350F (175C). Butter a 2½ quart casserole dish.

Cut a small cross in the stem of each sprout. Cook the sprouts in a large pot of boiling salted water until they are tender, about 8 minutes. Drain and rinse in cool water. Cut the sprouts in half; set aside.

Heat the butter and oil in a medium nonstick saucepan over medium heat and sauté the shallots until they are softened, about 3 minutes. Stir in the flour and cook over very low heat, stirring constantly, 3 minutes. Add the hot milk and whisk the sauce until it's smooth. Cook over medium-high heat, stirring constantly, until the mixture bubbles and thickens. Stir in the cheese and pepper and remove from the heat. Whisk occasionally while the heat of the sauce melts the cheese. Stir in the sprouts.

Spoon the rice into the prepared casserole dish, stirring in a few tablespoons of the sauce. Spoon the sprouts and the rest of the sauce on top and sprinkle with crumbs. Bake until golden on top and heated through, 25 to 30 minutes (40 to 45 if made ahead and refrigerated).

Makes 4 servings.

Baked Tomatoes Genovese

A lovely, light first course or side dish.

6 large ripe tomatoes
1 cup cooked brown rice, a little undercooked
1 tablespoon olive oil, plus more for drizzling
2 anchovy fillets, rinsed and chopped
2 tablespoons chopped pitted ripe olives
2 tablespoons finely diced pimiento or roasted red bell pepper
   (page 155)
2 tablespoons minced scallions
½ tablespoon minced fresh basil leaves or ½ teaspoon dried
   Freshly ground black pepper

Preheat the oven to 375F (190C).

Cut a ¼-inch slice off the stem ends of the tomatoes and reserve tops. Scoop out the seeds and pulp. Place the tomatoes upside down on paper towels to drain. Discard the seeds and chop the pulp. Mix the pulp (about 1 cup) with the rice and remaining ingredients, seasoning with pepper to taste.

Stuff the tomatoes with the rice mixture, and stand them in a baking dish that will hold them upright. Drizzle a little more olive oil over each tomato, and replace the tops as lids. Bake 30 minutes or until the tomatoes are soft but still hold their shape.

Serve at room temperature as an appetizer or side dish.

Makes 6 servings.

Sweet-and-Sour Maple Rutabaga

It's easier to peel a rutabaga if you first cut it in half, lay the halves cut sides down, slice them into 1-inch half-rounds, and then peel the rounds.

¾ pound rutabaga, peeled and diced (about 3 cups)
3 tablespoons pure maple syrup
2 tablespoons cider vinegar
 Salt

Cook the rutabaga in a saucepan over medium heat with water to cover. Simmer until the rutabaga is tender but not mushy, about 15 minutes. Drain. Toss the rutabaga with the maple syrup and vinegar. Add salt to taste. Cook, stirring constantly, over medium-high heat until the vinegar evaporates and rutabaga is slightly glazed.
Makes 4 servings.

Mashed Rutabagas and Apples

Rutabaga is a good source of indoles, phytochemicals that protect against many common cancers.

1 pound rutabagas, peeled and diced
2 apples, peeled and diced (Rome, Gala, or Macoun, not Delicious)
1 tablespoon butter
2 tablespoons honey
¼ teaspoon ground cinnamon

Cook the rutabagas in a large saucepan in boiling salted water to cover, until nearly tender, about 15 minutes. Add the apples and cook until both are tender, 5 minutes longer. Drain and mash the rutabagas and apples. Blend in the butter, honey, and cinnamon and serve warm.
Makes 4 servings.

Zucchini at the Savoy

Zucchini won't absorb much oil, and yet it does take on a much more interesting flavor when sautéed.

  1 medium-large (¾-lb.) zucchini
1½ tablespoons olive oil
  1 garlic clove, chopped
 ½ pound savoy cabbage, coarsely shredded
     Salt and freshly ground black pepper
  1 to 2 tablespoons balsamic vinegar (optional)

Trim off the ends of the zucchini and cut it slightly on the diagonal into ½-inch slices. Heat the oil in a 12-inch nonstick skillet over medium heat and lay the slices in it in one layer. Sauté the zucchini until it's lightly brown on one side. Turn the slices, scatter the garlic around them, and spread the cabbage on top. Cook until the cabbage begins to wilt, about 3 minutes. Stir-fry (turn the cabbage under the zucchini) until the cabbage is crisp-tender, 3 minutes more. Season with salt and pepper to taste. If desired, sprinkle with balsamic vinegar. Serve hot or at room temperature.

Makes 4 servings.

Spicy Summer Squash with Shelled Beans and Arborio Rice

This dish enlivens the blandness of summer squash with chiles.

  2 tablespoons olive oil
  2 fresh jalapeño chiles, seeded and minced (see Note, page 120)
 ½ cup chopped onion
  1 large garlic clove, minced
  2 cups canned tomatoes with juice
 ¼ teaspoon dried oregano
 ¼ teaspoon dried cilantro
 ¼ teaspoon salt
  1 pound fresh shell beans, shelled, or 1½ cups drained, rinsed, canned shell beans
  1 small summer squash, sliced into half-rounds
  2 cups cooked Arborio rice

Heat the oil in a large skillet over medium heat and sauté the chiles until slightly softened. Add the onion and garlic and sauté until they are sizzling. Add the tomatoes, herbs, salt, and fresh beans and simmer until the beans are almost tender, 15 minutes. (If using canned beans, simmer the sauce until thickened, 10 minutes, then add the beans.) Add the summer squash, and cook until the vegetables are quite tender, 5 to 7 minutes.

Spread the hot rice on a medium platter and spoon the vegetables and sauce over rice.

Makes 4 servings.

Early Summer Sauté

Substitute as you wish. Any small new vegetables may be cooked in this manner.

1   pound small new potatoes, unpeeled and halved
½   pound baby carrots, pared
½   pound young green beans
½   pound baby zucchini, quartered lengthwise
1   tablespoon olive oil
1   tablespoon butter
1   bunch scallions, cut into 1-inch lengths
    Salt and freshly ground black pepper

Bring a large pot of salted water to a boil for parboiling the vegetables. Cook them separately until just tender, about 10 minutes for the potatoes, 8 minutes for the carrots, and 5 minutes for the green beans. Remove with a slotted spoon and drain well. Do not parboil the zucchini.

Heat the oil and butter in a large skillet over medium heat and sauté the scallions until they are sizzling. Add the potatoes and zucchini and cook until the zucchini is nearly tender, 4 to 5 minutes. Add the carrots and green beans, and stir-fry until the vegetables begin to brown in places, about 10 minutes. Season with salt and pepper to taste.

Make 6 servings.

Fresh Succotash with Sun-Dried Tomatoes and Sage

The Mediterranean approach to a Native American dish.

1 tablespoon olive oil
1 large shallot, chopped
½ red bell pepper, diced
1 pound fresh shell beans, shelled (about 1½ cups shelled)
1 to 1½ cups Chicken-Mushroom Stock (page 333), Vegetable Stock
   (page 331), or canned broth
¼ teaspoon salt
⅛ teaspoon freshly ground pepper
   Corn kernels cut from 2 ears of fresh corn
6 sun-dried tomatoes (oil-packed), drained and diced
4 leaves fresh sage, chopped

Heat the oil in a heavy saucepan over medium heat and sauté the shallot and bell pepper until sizzling. Add the shelled beans and enough stock to almost cover them. Bring to a boil, reduce heat, and simmer, covered, until the beans are tender, 20 to 30 minutes. Season the beans with salt and pepper.

Stir in the corn and sun-dried tomatoes. Simmer 5 minutes or until corn is tender. Add the fresh sage, and cook 1 minute more. Serve in bowls.

Makes 4 servings.

Roasted Vegetable Pie with Polenta Topping

This savory combination makes a substantial and attractive vegetarian entree. It can also be served as a side dish with a meat entree, in which case portions would be smaller.

3½ cups Make-It-Easy Polenta (page 326)
  1 green bell pepper, seeded and cut into chunks
  1 mild green chile, seeded and cut into chunks
  4 plum tomatoes, quartered
  2 large potatoes, cut into 1-inch chunks
 ½ pound rutabaga, peeled and diced, or butternut squash, peeled and cut into chunks
  1 leek, rinsed and chopped
  5 ounces button mushrooms, cleaned
  2 tablespoons olive oil
  2 teaspoons minced fresh thyme or ½ teaspoon dried
  1 teaspoon chopped fresh rosemary or ¼ teaspoon dried
    Salt and freshly ground black pepper
  1 cup fresh shelled or frozen green peas
  2 tablespoons cornstarch
  3 tablespoons nonfat dry milk
  2 cups Vegetable Stock (page 331) or canned broth
 ¼ cup chopped fresh cilantro
  2 tablespoons freshly grated Parmesan cheese

Prepare the polenta in advance. Spoon it into an oiled 11 × 7-inch pan, and chill until it's firm. Cut the polenta into 8 squares.

Preheat the oven to 400F (205C). Toss the bell pepper, chile, tomatoes, potatoes, rutabaga, leek, and mushrooms with the oil, thyme, and rosemary, and put them into a large gratin pan or a nonreactive 13 × 9-inch baking dish. Salt and pepper them to taste. Roast the vegetables until they are tender, 45 to 50 minutes. Remove the vegetables from the oven and stir in the peas. Reduce oven temperature to 350F (175C).

Meanwhile, make the sauce. Stir the cornstarch and dry milk into the stock in a medium saucepan until blended. Bring to a boil, stirring constantly, until the sauce bubbles and thickens. Reduce the heat and simmer, stirring occasionally, 5 minutes. Stir in the cilantro. Taste to correct seasoning, adding salt if needed. (Remember that the sauce will pick up the seasonings in the vegetables.) Pour the sauce over the vegetables.

Layer the polenta on top, overlapping slices if necessary. Sprinkle with the cheese. (The dish can be prepared ahead to this point and refrigerated several hours until ready to cook.)

Bake the dish until the filling is bubbling and the polenta is lightly colored, 20 to 25 minutes (30 to 40 minutes if the dish has been prepared ahead and refrigerated).

Makes 4 main-dish servings.

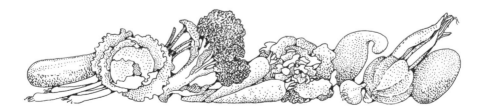

Grilled Vegetables with Balsamic Vinegar

If your grill isn't up and running, you can broil the vegetables, 6 inches from the heat source, which takes about 15 minutes. The result is similar, minus the smoky flavor.

¼ cup olive oil
 1 garlic clove, quartered
½ teaspoon salt
¼ teaspoon freshly ground black pepper
 2 red bell peppers, seeded and quartered lengthwise
 2 green bell peppers, seeded and quartered lengthwise
 4 large green onions, quartered
 1 medium zucchini, quartered lengthwise
 4 baby eggplant, unpeeled and halved lengthwise
 2 tablespoons balsamic vinegar

Prepare the grill. Position a rack 6 inches from heat.

Mix the oil, garlic, salt, and black pepper in a wide, shallow dish. Add the vegetables and marinate 20 minutes, tossing occasionally. Drain, reserving any remaining oil.

Grill the vegetables until tender, about 10 minutes for the bell peppers and zucchini, and 15 minutes for the eggplant. Transfer to a platter. If desired, brush them with the reserved marinade. Sprinkle with the vinegar. Serve warm or at room temperature.

Makes 4 servings.

Four-C Vegetable Stir-Fry

Cauliflower, carrots, cabbage, and cashews combine in a stir-fry that's rich in phytochemicals to promote immunity.

1½ cups Vegetable Stock (page 331) or canned broth
  1 tablespoon naturally brewed soy sauce, plus more to pass
  1 teaspoon sesame oil
  4 teaspoons cornstarch
  1 teaspoon brown sugar
¼ teaspoon cayenne pepper
  2 tablespoons canola oil
  2 cups cauliflower flowerets, sliced about ½ inch thick
  1 cup very thin carrot slices
  1 bunch scallions, sliced diagonally into 1-inch pieces
  2 slices fresh ginger, peeled and minced
  3 cups shredded Napa or green cabbage
  1 garlic clove, minced
½ cup cashews
    Hot cooked rice, brown or white

Combine the stock, soy sauce, sesame oil, cornstarch, sugar, and cayenne in a saucepan, whisking to blend and dissolve the cornstarch. Bring to a boil, stirring constantly. Reduce heat and simmer about 2 minutes, stirring occasionally.

Heat the oil in a large wok or skillet. Add the cauliflower, carrots, scallions, and ginger and stir-fry until vegetables are nearly crisp-tender, 3 to 5 minutes. Add the cabbage and garlic and stir-fry until the cabbage is wilted and crisp-tender, about 2 minutes more. Add the sauce and heat through.

Transfer the vegetables to a serving dish and sprinkle with the cashews. Serve with hot rice on the side. Pass soy sauce at the table.

Makes 4 servings.

Greens 'n' Beans Gumbo

When you make this dish, it's nice to have a "gumbo buddy" in the kitchen to help stir the roux. Alternatively, you can make the roux as much as a week ahead and keep it refrigerated until needed.

  3 tablespoons canola oil
¼ cup unbleached all-purpose flour
  1 green bell pepper, diced
  1 large yellow onion, diced
  1 celery stalk, diced
  2 garlic cloves, minced
  1 (14- to 16-oz.) can plum tomatoes with juice
½ cup water
⅓ pound fresh okra, trimmed and sliced
  1 (16-oz.) can red kidney beans, drained and rinsed, or 2 cups
     cooked (page 328)
½ pound mustard or turnip greens, tough stems removed, chopped
  1 teaspoon hot pepper sauce
½ teaspoon dried thyme
¼ teaspoon cayenne pepper
⅛ teaspoon freshly ground black pepper
¼ teaspoon salt
1½ cups fresh or frozen whole-kernel corn
  3 cups hot cooked white rice

Blend the oil and flour in a large heavy pot over medium-low heat and cook, stirring very often, until dark golden brown, 20 to 30 minutes. At first the mixture will be lumpy, but as it cooks and changes color, it becomes creamy. Don't settle for light brown; go for mahogany, but don't burn the roux.

Stir the bell pepper, onion, and celery into the roux, and cook over low heat until the vegetables begin to soften, 5 to 8 minutes. Add the garlic and cook 1 minute. Add the tomatoes, water, okra, beans, greens, hot pepper sauce, thyme, cayenne pepper, black pepper, and salt. Simmer, covered, stirring often, 20 to 25 minutes, until okra is tender and the mixture is thick and flavorful. Add the corn and cook 5 minutes more. Taste to correct seasoning, adding more salt or hot pepper sauce as desired.

Serve the gumbo in large soup plates with a spoonful of rice in the center.

Makes 6 servings.

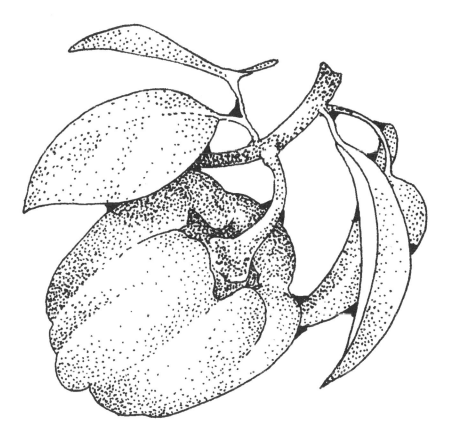

Mashed Root-Vegetable Medley

Lots of vitamin A for protection against winter woes.

1½ pounds sweet potatoes, peeled and cut into 1-inch pieces
1½ pounds russet potatoes, peeled and cut into 1-inch pieces
  1 pound rutabagas, peeled and cut into ½-inch pieces
  ¾ teaspoon salt
  2 tablespoons butter, melted
  1 cup plain nonfat yogurt
  ¼ teaspoon white pepper
  2 tablespoons chopped fresh chives or minced scallion tops, or
    1 tablespoon freeze-dried chives

Combine the vegetables, ½ teaspoon of the salt, and enough water to cover in a large saucepan. Bring to a boil, cover, and simmer until everything is quite tender, about 25 minutes.

Drain and mash the vegetables. Whisk in the remaining ¼ teaspoon salt, butter, yogurt, white pepper, and chives. Beat until fluffy. (A hand-held electric mixer makes this task easier.)

Serve immediately.

Makes 6 servings.

NOTE

To make up to 1 day ahead, transfer mashed vegetables to a buttered casserole dish, cover and refrigerate. Reheat, covered, in a preheated 350F (175C) oven 30 minutes. Uncover and bake another 5 to 10 minutes, until golden on top.

Stir-Fried Vegetables with Tofu and Pineapple

Tofu, shiitakes, and some super vegetables make this dish a great immune-system booster. As with any stir-fry, it's best to have all the ingredients (and the rice) prepared before beginning to cook. The actual cooking time is only 5 minutes or so.

2   tablespoons vegetable oil
1   carrot, very thinly sliced
1   small turnip, peeled and thinly sliced
2   slices fresh ginger, minced
4   scallions, chopped
2   celery stalks, very thinly sliced
4   fresh shiitake mushrooms, stems removed (discard or save for stock), slivered
1   red bell pepper, seeded and cut into small triangles
2   cups fresh spinach, shredded
½   pound firm tofu, diced
1   cup fresh pineapple chunks or canned, drained chunks
2   tablespoons naturally brewed soy sauce
2   teaspoons oyster sauce
4   cups hot cooked brown or white rice

Heat 1 tablespoon of the oil in a large wok or skillet over high heat and stir-fry the carrot, turnip, and ginger 1 minute. Add the scallions, celery, mushrooms, and bell pepper. Add the remaining 1 tablespoon of oil, if needed, and stir-fry until the carrot and turnip are almost crisp-tender, 1 to 2 minutes more. Add the spinach, tofu, and pineapple, and cook, stirring, until the spinach has wilted, 1 to 2 minutes. Season with soy sauce and oyster sauce. Serve with hot rice.

Makes 4 servings.

Zesty Tofu-Bean Chili

Quick, easy, and fun to eat.

   2 tablespoons olive oil
   1 large yellow onion, chopped
   2 garlic cloves, minced
1½ tablespoons chili powder
   1 teaspoon ground cumin
   1 teaspoon ground coriander
   ½ teaspoon anise seeds
   1 (15- to 16-oz.) can tomatoes
   1 (14- to 16-oz.) can pinto beans, drained and rinsed, or 2 cups
       cooked (page 328)
   1 yellow bell pepper, seeded and diced
   2 fresh or canned jalapeño chiles, seeded and minced (see Note,
       page 120)
   1 (14-oz.) package firm tofu, diced
   ⅛ teaspoon cayenne pepper or to taste

   Accompaniments
   ½ cup plain nonfat yogurt
    2 scallions, finely chopped
    1 small ripe avocado
       Juice of ½ lime plus 4 lime wedges
    1 cup (4 oz.) shredded Monterey Jack cheese
       Baked tortilla chips

   Heat the oil in a Dutch oven or other large heavy pan over medium heat and sauté the onion until softened, about 5 minutes. Stir in the garlic, chili powder, cumin, coriander, and anise seeds and cook over very low heat, stirring, 1 to 2 minutes, until quite fragrant. Add the tomatoes, beans, bell pepper, and chiles and simmer, covered, 20 minutes. Gently stir in the tofu and simmer, with cover ajar, 5 minutes. Add cayenne to taste, starting with ⅛ teaspoon. Cook 1 minute, and taste again, adding more if desired.

Prepare the accompaniments: Mix the yogurt with the minced scallions. Dice the avocado and stir in the juice of ½ lime. Serve the chili with yogurt mixture, avocado, lime wedges, shredded cheese, and tortilla chips, each in a separate dish.

Makes 4 servings.

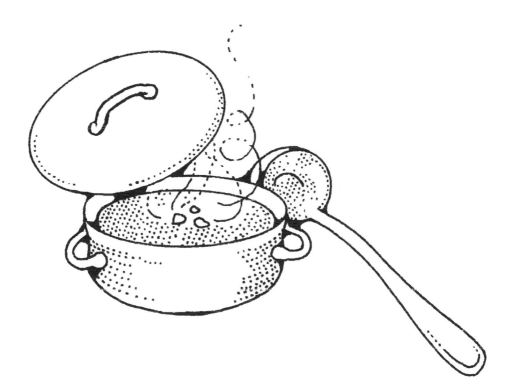

Super Salads Every Day—
and Here's Why

Gone are the days when "salad" meant a wedge of iceberg lettuce with a vaguely orange dressing poured over it or a shimmering square of sweet gelatin with a surprising conglomeration of ingredients. Salads today are big, bold, and inventive. Although most of them are cool and crunchy, some of the newest may include cooked or even warm ingredients. Some are simple and artful; others are a marvelous medley of vegetables or fruits. Either way, they offer a host of vitamins, minerals, and phytochemicals. Raw food does have a slight nutritional edge over cooked food, because cooking can diminish heat-sensitive nutrients—vitamin C and the B vitamins. Of the phytochemicals, sulforaphane has proved to be unaffected by cooking; others have yet to be studied.

A chilled salad made with raw foods provides a welcome counterpoint to cooked foods served at the same meal. Menus simply seem to balance better, in taste as well as nutrition, when a salad is included. Many of today's salad dressings are oil-based vinaigrettes made with olive, nut, or seed oils that are actually good for you (in moderation), because they are the best source of that elusive heart-saver, vitamin E. Linoleic (LA) and alpha linolenic (LNA) acids, which salad oils provide, are essential to the brain's capacity to learn.

The American custom is to serve the salad course first. In the Mediterranean region, however, salads are served as a "refresher" after

251

the entree. Whichever style you prefer, a well-designed salad rounds out the main meal of the day with a big helping of good nutrition.

But it's not just a dinner dish. A salad is the quintessential light lunch, provided it's not drowned in creamy dressing. Preparing a salad for lunch may seem like a lot more trouble than slapping together a fast sandwich, but *you're worth it*. Getting a number of salad ingredients ready before they are needed is an encouraging time-saver. Think of your refrigerator as a mini–salad bar in which you stash items like chopped scallions, shredded carrots, sliced celery, marinated artichokes, roasted peppers, raw cauliflowerets, bell pepper rings, crumbled cheese, and a bag of washed, spun-dry greens wrapped in a kitchen towel and a plastic bag. A batch of these mix-and-match salad ingredients will keep in the refrigerator for three to four days.

A word about salad greens: Never in our history have we had so many from which to choose—green or red leafy lettuce, frisée, tender young spinach, chicory, radicchio, romaine, escarole (inner leaves), arugula, watercress, and, yes, good old iceberg lettuce. Enjoy them all!

Green Salad with Kiwifruit and Shaved Parmesan

Kiwifruit adds a sweet-tart touch of glamour to this mixed-green salad.

- 6 cups rinsed, spun-dry, bite-size mixed greens, such as tender baby spinach, frisée, romaine, red leaf lettuce, watercress
- 1 cup shredded radicchio
- 4 kiwifruit, peeled and sliced
- ½ cup loosely packed, shaved Parmesan cheese
- 3 tablespoons extra-virgin olive oil
- 2 to 3 tablespoons red wine vinegar
  Salt and freshly ground black pepper

Arrange the greens in a large salad bowl. Sprinkle with radicchio. Lay the kiwi slices on top. Scatter the Parmesan cheese over all.

When ready to serve, dress with oil and vinegar. Add salt and pepper to taste. Toss gently to combine.

Makes 6 servings.

Medley of Greens with Light Blue Cheese Dressing

If you love blue cheese dressing but fear the fat, here's a light version my family enjoys.

1 red onion, thinly sliced and separated into rings
2 cups bite-size romaine lettuce
2 cups bite-size tender spinach, stems removed
2 cups bite-size red leaf lettuce

Light Blue Cheese Dressing
1 teaspoon chopped fresh dill or ¼ teaspoon dried
¼ teaspoon dry mustard
¼ teaspoon celery salt
¼ teaspoon white pepper
1 cup nonfat plain yogurt
½ cup crumbled blue cheese

Soak the onion rings in ice water about 30 minutes to sweeten them. Drain and combine the onion rings and salad greens in a bowl.

Prepare the dressing: Blend the dill, mustard, celery salt, and pepper into the yogurt in a small bowl. Stir in the blue cheese.

Serve the salad with the dressing on the side. Leftover dressing may be kept refrigerated up to a week.

Makes 4 servings.

Bundles-of-Asparagus Salad with Prosciutto

This attractive and versatile salad can be served as an antipasto or first course, as a luncheon dish, or as an accompaniment to a summer entree, such as cold poached salmon.

1   pound fresh asparagus with very thin stalks
    Inner leaves of romaine lettuce
8   slices (about ⅛ lb.) prosciutto
1 to 2 whole roasted oil-packed bell peppers from a jar, drained and
    cut into 8 strips
4   teaspoons red wine vinegar
    About 3 tablespoons extra-virgin olive oil
    Freshly ground black pepper

Trim off the woody ends of the asparagus and rinse the stalks well. Lay them in a large skillet with about ½ inch salted water and bring to a boil. Cover and reduce heat. Cook until crisp-tender, 2 to 3 minutes for thin stalks. Drain and rinse in cold water (in the skillet is the easiest way) until the stalks are no longer warm. Drain again. Chill the asparagus.

Arrange lettuce leaves, torn into thirds, on 4 large salad plates. Divide the asparagus into 8 bundles. Wrap each bundle in a slice of prosciutto and a strip of roasted pepper. Lay 2 bundles on each plate. Sprinkle each salad with a teaspoon of vinegar and about 2 teaspoons of oil. Season with freshly ground pepper.

Makes 4 servings.

Three-Bean Salad for the Nineties

A fresh new version of the old church-supper favorite.

½ pound fresh green beans
½ pound fresh yellow wax beans
1½ pounds fresh cranberry beans, shelled (about 2 cups) or 1 (14- to 16-oz.) can pinto or pink beans, drained and rinsed
1 tablespoon minced fresh basil or 1 teaspoon dried
1 tablespoon minced fresh cilantro or 1 teaspoon dried
3 tablespoons olive oil
2 tablespoons white wine vinegar
¼ teaspoon *each* sugar and salt
⅛ teaspoon white pepper
1 large ripe tomato or 2 plum tomatoes, seeded and diced
4 scallions with green tops, chopped
Last-Minute Garlic Bread (opposite)

Trim the ends from the green and yellow beans. Cook the green beans in a large pot of salted boiling water until tender, about 5 minutes. Remove with a slotted spoon and rinse in cold water. Cook the yellow beans in the same water until tender, about 3 minutes. Finally, cook the cranberry beans, about 15 minutes, drain and rinse. If desired, chill the vegetables until ready to compose the salad.

Combine the herbs, oil, vinegar, sugar, salt, and pepper in a salad bowl and whisk to dissolve the sugar and to blend well. Stir in the tomato, scallions, and all the beans. Let the salad marinate at room temperature about 30 minutes before serving with Last-Minute Garlic Bread.

Makes 6 to 8 servings.

Last-Minute Garlic Bread

Quick and easy, this bread complements almost any salad or soup.

16 slices French bread
 1 garlic clove, halved
    Extra-virgin olive oil
    Freshly grated Parmesan cheese
    Dried oregano

Preheat broiler. Gently but thoroughly rub both sides of the slices with the cut clove of garlic. Toast the slices on one side under preheated broiler until just golden, about 3 minutes. Turn and drizzle a little olive oil on each slice. Sprinkle with cheese and oregano. Toast the second side about 3 minutes.

Makes 8 servings.

Green Beans with Walnut and Dill Dressing

Add the vinegar just before serving to preserve the bright color of the greens. Walnut oil, once opened, should be stored in the refrigerator. Fresh dill is preferred, if available.

1 pound fresh whole green beans, ends trimmed
2 tablespoons walnut oil
1 tablespoon minced fresh dill or 1 teaspoon dried dill
¼ teaspoon salt
⅛ teaspoon freshly ground black pepper
4 scallions, chopped
2 tablespoons white wine vinegar
⅓ cup walnut halves or pieces
½ cup finely diced Gruyère or Swiss cheese

Cook the green beans in boiling salted water until they are crisp-tender, about 5 minutes. Drain and rinse in cold water. Shake off excess water or blot dry with paper towels.

Toss the green beans with the walnut oil, dill, salt, pepper, and scallions. Chill until ready to serve. Add the wine vinegar, walnuts, and cheese, and toss again.

Makes 4 servings.

Tossed Greens 'n' Beans Salad

Add beans to salad for a boost of protein for energy, B vitamins for your nerves, calcium for your bones, and phytochemicals for protection—what a great bonus! If soybeans are not in your local supermarket, try a natural foods store.

    2 tablespoons red wine vinegar
    3 tablespoons olive oil
    1 tablespoon snipped fresh herbs: basil, marjoram, parsley,
      savory, and/or chives
    ¼ teaspoon salt (optional)
      Freshly ground black pepper
    1 cup canned soybeans or chick-peas, drained and rinsed, or
      1 cup cooked (page 328)
    1 large ripe tomato, diced
    2 to 3 inner celery stalks with leaves, finely chopped
    ¼ cup chopped red onion
    ½ cup diced fresh cheese: feta, ricotta salata, or mozzarella
    4 cups rinsed, spun-dry mixed greens: romaine, leaf lettuce, chicory,
      frisée, escarole (inner leaves), or watercress—choose at least 2
      kinds

Combine the vinegar, oil, herbs, salt, and pepper to taste in a large salad bowl. Add the soybeans, tomato, celery, onion, and cheese and toss lightly.

Arrange the greens on top of other ingredients without tossing and refrigerate the salad on the bottom shelf, covered with a kitchen towel, until ready to serve. The greens will be crisp and the vegetables marinated. Toss well just before serving.

Makes 4 servings.

Pickled Baked Beets

Beets take on a different, more earthy flavor when baked.

2 pounds (4 to 6 large) beets
½ cup cider vinegar
¼ cup water
¼ cup sugar
½ teaspoon celery salt
1 small yellow onion, thinly sliced
1 tablespoon chopped fresh dill or 1 teaspoon dried
¼ teaspoon freshly ground black pepper

Preheat the oven to 325F (165C).

Scrub the beets, but don't peel them. Wrap each one in foil. Place them in a baking pan and bake until tender, 1¼ to 2 hours. Peel back the foil to test, using the point of a paring knife. Unwrap and cool the beets.

Peel and slice the beets into thin rounds and put them into a deep medium bowl. Combine the vinegar, water, sugar, and celery salt in a small saucepan. Heat, stirring, just long enough to dissolve the sugar and salt. Remove from the heat and add the onion, dill, and pepper. Stir vinegar mixture into the beets. Chill the salad, covered, for several hours or overnight before serving.

Makes 6 servings.

VARIATION

Chicory and Beet Salad

Follow the preceding recipe. Line a salad bowl with 4 cups crisp, chopped chicory and spoon the beets on top, leaving a margin of green around the sides. Serve with bakery-fresh crusty rye bread.

Cauliflower and Roasted Pepper Salad

Cauliflower cooked just until tender is much sweeter. Longer cooking brings out a strong flavor (and smells up the kitchen).

 1 large red bell pepper
 1 large green bell pepper
 4 tablespoons extra-virgin olive oil
 1 garlic clove, peeled and halved
    Salt and freshly ground pepper
 2 cups cooked, crisp-tender cauliflowerets (cooked about 3 minutes)
 1 tablespoon drained capers
 ¼ cup chopped red onion
 ¼ cup chopped celery tops and leaves
 4 cups mixed salad greens, in bite-size pieces
 3 tablespoons fresh lemon juice

A few hours before making the salad, prepare and marinate the bell peppers: Roast and peel the bell peppers according to directions on page 155 and cut them into strips. Place them in a bowl, add 2 tablespoons of the oil and the garlic, and season with salt and pepper to taste. Allow them to marinate at room temperature about 30 minutes. When ready to assemble the salad, remove the garlic.

Toss together the cauliflower, peppers, capers, onion, celery, and greens in a large salad bowl. Drizzle on the lemon juice and remaining 2 tablespoons of oil. Season with salt and pepper to taste. Serve immediately.

Makes 4 servings.

Tomato and Parsley Salad with
Roasted-Garlic Vinaigrette

Serve a crusty Mediterranean bread on the side to dip in the salad juices and voilá—instant garlic bread.

 4 garlic cloves (see Note below)
 ¼ cup olive oil
 3 tablespoons red wine vinegar
 ¼ teaspoon salt
 ⅛ teaspoon freshly ground black pepper
 6 medium ripe tomatoes, sliced
 ½ cup chopped fresh flat-leaf parsley

Preheat the oven to 375F (190C). Cut off the tops of the garlic cloves and wrap them in foil. Bake 45 minutes or until soft when pressed. Cool the garlic enough to handle. Squeeze the garlic cloves out of their skins.

Mash the garlic with the oil. Whisk in vinegar, salt, and pepper. Arrange the tomatoes on a platter. Scatter the parsley on top. Pour the dressing over all. Let stand at room temperature 15 to 20 minutes before serving.

Makes 4 servings.

NOTE
Instead of 4 cloves, you can roast a whole bulb, if you plan to use the rest in another dish. Follow the same directions. Refrigerate extra garlic.

Layered Tomato, Mozzarella, and Basil Salad

This is a nice light salad to include in an appetizer buffet. It disappears quickly, so it's best to have a backup platter in the kitchen. Preparation couldn't be simpler, but the quality of the ingredients is essential—no substitutes!

8 medium, vine-ripened tomatoes, sliced
   About 40 fresh whole basil leaves
2 (½-lb. each) fresh whole-milk or part-skim mozzarella cheese balls,
   sliced into half-rounds
   Salt and freshly ground black pepper
⅓ cup extra-virgin olive oil
1 thin loaf French bread

On a large platter, alternate slices of tomato with fresh whole basil leaves and half-rounds of mozzarella cheese. Season with salt and pepper to taste and drizzle with the oil.

Serve with a basket of sliced French bread on the side.

Makes 8 servings.

Yellow Tomato Salad with Red Onion and Arugula

Yellow tomatoes are slightly less acidic than red ones. If you grow tomatoes, this is a fun vegetable to add to your garden and, since they are expensive to buy, a worthwhile effort.

1 medium red onion, sliced and separated into rings (use only large outer rings; save the rest for another use)
4 yellow tomatoes, sliced
  Salt and freshly ground black pepper
3 tablespoons extra-virgin olive oil
1 tablespoon white wine vinegar
1 bunch arugula or watercress, rinsed, stemmed, and chopped

Soak the onion rings in ice water 30 minutes or so to sweeten them. Drain.

Lay the tomato slices and onion rings in a flat serving dish with a rim. Salt and pepper them to taste, and drizzle with olive oil and vinegar. Let stand at room temperature 15 minutes.

Before serving, add the arugula and toss gently. Taste a leaf to see if you want more oil or vinegar.

Makes 4 servings.

Tomato and Fresh Pineapple Salad

A great "go-along" with grilled meats! Choosing a ripe but not over-ripe pineapple is a tricky proposition. Rather than relying on the ease with which a leaf can be pulled from the pineapple top, I like to choose the fruit with the best pineapple aroma. There should be no hint of a winelike fragrance, however; that would mean the fruit has begun to decline. Some supermarkets sell ready-peeled pineapples in plastic containers—a great convenience.

4 large ripe tomatoes, sliced
1 fresh ripe pineapple, peeled, cored, and sliced
½ cup chopped green onions, preferably sweet onions
¼ cup extra-virgin olive oil
  Salt
  Freshly ground black pepper

Alternate slices of tomato and pineapple on a platter. Sprinkle with green onions. Drizzle with olive oil. Season with salt to taste and a lot of black pepper. Let stand at room temperature 15 minutes before serving.
Makes 6 servings.

Braised Brussels Sprout and Carrot Salad with Balsamic Vinegar

Braising with shallots gives these vegetables an incomparable flavor.

½ pound carrots, sliced diagonally into 1-inch pieces
1 pint fresh brussels sprouts or 1 (10-oz.) package frozen brussels sprouts
2 tablespoons olive oil
½ cup sliced shallots
1 teaspoon minced fresh tarragon or ¼ teaspoon dried
Salt and freshly ground black pepper
2 tablespoons balsamic vinegar

Parboil the carrots in salted water 5 minutes; drain. Clean the sprouts and cut an × in the root end. Parboil until crisp-tender, about 8 minutes. Or cook frozen sprouts according to package directions. Drain and cut the sprouts in half.

Heat 1 tablespoon oil in a large skillet over medium heat and stir-fry the vegetables with the shallots until they are lightly browned, 5 minutes. Transfer to a serving bowl. Toss with tarragon, salt and pepper to taste, the remaining 1 tablespoon of oil, and the vinegar. Serve at room temperature.

Makes 4 servings.

Asian Vegetable Salad

Both radishes and bok choy are cancer-fighting cruciferous vegetables.

½ pound fresh snow peas
 4 large stalks bok choy, thinly sliced, or 2 cups shredded
    napa cabbage
 1 cup thinly sliced radishes
1½ cups fresh bean sprouts, rinsed
½ cup chopped scallion tops

Dressing
 3 tablespoons unseasoned rice vinegar
 3 tablespoons peanut or canola oil
 1 teaspoon sesame oil
½ teaspoon sugar
¼ teaspoon salt
 1 slice fresh ginger very finely minced or ½ teaspoon ground ginger

Trim and string the snow peas. Cook them in boiling salted water 1 minute, counting from the time the bubbling resumes. Drain and rinse the snow peas in cold water.

Combine the vegetables in a large salad bowl.

Mix the dressing ingredients together in a jar. Cover and shake to blend. Pour the dressing over the salad and toss well. Chill the salad until ready to serve. Taste to correct the seasoning; you may want more vinegar.

Makes 4 servings.

Italian Potato Salad with Artichoke Hearts

This vinaigrette-dressed potato salad keeps well and is a good choice for a picnic. If the onion is too strong for your taste, soak it in ice water for 15 to 20 minutes, then drain and chop.

3   pounds red potatoes, scrubbed
1   teaspoon salt
1   tablespoon white wine vinegar
½   cup finely chopped red onion
¾   cup Vinaigrette (page 337)
½   teaspoon dried oregano
     Freshly ground black pepper
2   (14-oz.) cans artichoke hearts, drained
½   cup finely chopped fresh flat-leaf parsley

Cut the potatoes into uniform size—halves or quarters—and steam them over water to which you've added the salt and vinegar, until tender but not mushy, 10 to 15 minutes. Cool the potatoes until they can be handled. Peel and dice them into a large bowl. Toss with the chopped onion, ½ cup of the vinaigrette, oregano, and pepper to taste. Cut the artichoke hearts in half, and gently stir them into the salad. Chill.

When ready to serve, toss the salad again, adding ¼ cup or more of the remaining vinaigrette and the parsley.

Makes 8 servings.

Hussar's Salad

Originally Russian, this hearty salad was adopted by the Dutch and became quite a favorite buffet dish. Although this is a vegetable version, for a heartier (and more traditional) salad, stir in 2 cups diced cold meat—veal, turkey, chicken, or any roast—and serve it as a main dish. Fresh crusty rye bread is a perfect accompaniment.

3	medium potatoes (1 pound), peeled and diced
3	medium beets (½ pound), scrubbed
1	Granny Smith apple, peeled and diced
¼	cup chopped scallions
2	tablespoons chopped sweet pickles
2	tablespoons canola oil
2	tablespoons cider vinegar
¼	teaspoon salt
⅛	teaspoon freshly ground pepper
	Romaine lettuce leaves
3	large plum tomatoes, sliced
2	hard-cooked eggs, peeled and sliced
2	tablespoons mayonnaise
¼	cup nonfat plain yogurt
1	tablespoon chili sauce

Steam the potatoes until tender, about 12 minutes; cool. Cook unpeeled beets in a separate pot of boiling salted water until they are tender, 30 to 35 minutes. Cool, peel, and dice the beets.

Gently toss together the potatoes, beets, apple, scallions, pickles, oil, vinegar, salt, and pepper in a large bowl.

Arrange lettuce leaves on a large platter. Heap the potato mixture in the center and surround the salad with sliced tomatoes and eggs. Whisk together the mayonnaise, yogurt, and chili sauce. Spread or drizzle this dressing over the top. Chill the salad until ready to serve.

Makes 4 servings.

Potato and Asparagus Salad

This delicious eye-catching salad with lots of B vitamins is very easily assembled.

- 1 tablespoon olive oil
- 1 red bell pepper, seeded and cut into 2-inch sticks
- 1 garlic clove, minced
- 1 pound fresh asparagus, tough part of stems removed and stalks cut into 2-inch pieces
- 2 pounds potatoes, peeled and cut into 2-inch sticks (similar to french fries)
- ⅓ cup nonfat plain yogurt
- 2 tablespoons mayonnaise
  A few sprigs of fresh parsley, chopped
- ¼ teaspoon salt
- ¼ teaspoon white pepper
- 4 scallions, cut diagonally into 2-inch pieces

Heat the oil in a large skillet and sauté the bell pepper over medium heat until it's just crisp-tender, 3 minutes. Add the garlic and cook 1 minute. Remove the bell pepper and as much of the garlic as you can.

Wipe out the skillet, add ½ cup water and the asparagus, and simmer until it's crisp-tender, about 3 minutes.

Meanwhile, cook the potatoes separately in boiling salted water until tender, 5 to 7 minutes. Drain and cool the potatoes slightly.

Combine the yogurt, mayonnaise, parsley, salt, and white pepper in a small bowl. Combine the potatoes, asparagus, bell pepper, and scallions in a salad bowl. Blend in the yogurt mixture. Cover and chill until needed. Let stand at room temperature 10 to 15 minutes before serving.

Makes 6 servings.

Shelled Bean Salad with Walnuts

Walnuts should be added at the last minute, since they darken the salad if they marinate with the other ingredients.

1½ pounds fresh shell beans, shelled (about 2 cups) or
    1 (16-oz.) can shell or pinto beans, drained and rinsed
  1 celery stalk with leaves, diced
  1 small red bell pepper, seeded and diced
½ cup chopped red onion
  3 tablespoons walnut oil or olive oil
  2 tablespoons red wine vinegar
¼ teaspoon salt
¼ teaspoon freshly ground black pepper
  1 cup walnut halves or pieces
  1 tablespoon minced fresh flat-leaf parsley

Cook the shelled beans, if fresh, in boiling salted water to cover until tender, about 20 minutes. Drain and rinse to cool beans.

Combine all ingredients except walnuts and parsley in a serving dish and toss to blend. Cover and chill until ready to serve. Taste to correct seasoning, adding more oil, vinegar, salt, or pepper as desired. Toss with walnuts and parsley.

Makes 4 servings.

Corn Relish and Black Bean Salad

A great crowd-pleasing dish for a buffet.

2 cups fresh or frozen whole-kernel corn, cooked and cooled
1 (14- to 16-oz.) can black beans, drained and rinsed, or
   2 cups cooked (page 328)
1 red bell pepper, seeded and finely diced
1 green bell pepper, seeded and finely diced
½ cup chopped Vidalia or other sweet onion
1 to 2 fresh or canned jalapeño chiles, seeded and minced
   (see Note, page 120)
1 garlic clove, pressed through a garlic press
   Juice of 1 large lime (about 2 tablespoons)
2 tablespoons rice vinegar
2 tablespoons olive oil
¼ cup chopped fresh cilantro or flat-leaf parsley
½ teaspoon salt
⅛ to ¼ teaspoon freshly ground black pepper

Combine corn, beans, bell peppers, and onion in a large bowl. Mix in the chile and garlic until thoroughly blended with the other vegetables. Stir in the remaining ingredients. Cover and chill about 1 hour before serving. Toss well and taste to correct seasoning, adding more of the dressing ingredients or seasonings as you wish.

Makes 6 servings.

Lentil and Chopped Vegetable Salad

Leftovers make a wonderful lunch. Try this salad in a pita pocket for a vegetarian sandwich.

1 cup lentils, picked over and rinsed
3 cups water
1 garlic clove, crushed
   Salt
1 large tomato, diced
1 cup chopped fennel or celery
6 to 8 radishes, thinly sliced
1 large carrot, cut crosswise into paper-thin slices
4 scallions, chopped
3 tablespoons extra-virgin olive oil
2 tablespoons red wine vinegar
   Freshly ground black pepper
1 tablespoon minced fresh flat-leaf parsley

   Combine the lentils, water, garlic, and ½ teaspoon salt in a saucepan. Bring to a boil and simmer, uncovered, until the lentils are just tender but still retain their shape, 20 to 25 minutes. Drain and rinse in cool water. Discard the garlic.

   Mix together the lentils, tomato, fennel, radishes, carrot, and scallions in a salad bowl. Add the oil and vinegar with salt and pepper to taste. Stir in the parsley. Let the salad stand at room temperature 15 to 20 minutes before serving.

   Makes 4 servings.

Spicy Vegetable Tabbouleh

Tabbouleh is a Middle Eastern salad made with nutritious bulgur wheat. This version departs from the traditional by adding some zesty Mexican flavors.

> 2 cups Vegetable Stock (page 331), Chicken-Mushroom Stock (page 333), or canned broth
> 1 teaspoon ground cumin
> ¼ teaspoon salt
> ⅛ teaspoon cayenne pepper
> 1 cup bulgur
> 1½ cups fresh or frozen whole-kernel corn, cooked crisp-tender
> 1½ cups seeded, diced plum tomatoes
> 1 small green bell pepper, seeded and diced
> 4 scallions, finely chopped
> 1 garlic clove, pressed through a garlic press or very finely minced
> 1 jalapeño chile, fresh or canned, seeded and minced (see Note, page 120)
> 2 tablespoons minced fresh cilantro or 1 teaspoon dried
> 1 tablespoon minced fresh mint or ½ teaspoon dried
> ¼ cup olive oil
> 3 tablespoons fresh lime juice (about 1½ limes)

Bring the stock to a boil in a medium saucepan. Stir in the cumin, salt, cayenne, and bulgur. Remove from the heat, cover, and let stand until all the liquid is absorbed and the bulgur is cool. Fluff the grains with a fork.

Combine the bulgur, corn, tomatoes, bell pepper, and scallions in a salad bowl. Stir in the garlic and chile, taking care to distribute them evenly throughout the mixture. Dress the salad with cilantro, mint, olive oil, and lime juice. Toss, cover, and chill. Taste to correct seasoning, adding more salt, cayenne, oil, or lime juice, if desired.

Makes 4 servings.

Greek Garden Salad on Pita "Plates"

You can serve pita bread on the side, of course, but this way the bread catches all the lovely juices. If you want to make it easier to eat, cut the pita into wedges and re-form it into a round before topping with salad. Ricotta salata is a firm ricotta, much like feta cheese.

Dressing (see below)
4 scallions, thinly sliced
¼ cup chopped, pitted green Greek olives
½ pound plum tomatoes, thinly sliced
1 cucumber, peeled if waxed, thinly sliced
1 small head romaine lettuce, separated into leaves, washed, and spun dry
¼ cup crumbed feta cheese or ricotta salata
2 marinated artichoke hearts (optional), quartered
4 pita bread rounds

Dressing
1 cup olive oil
Juice of 2 lemons (½ cup), strained
1 teaspoon dried oregano
½ teaspoon salt
Freshly ground black pepper to taste

Prepare dressing: Combine the ingredients in a jar or bottle with a tight-fitting lid and shake well. This makes enough dressing for two or three salads. Shake before measuring.

Combine ⅓ cup of the dressing with the scallions, olives, tomatoes, and cucumber in a large salad bowl and toss them together.

Tear the romaine into bite-size pieces and arrange the romaine on top of the other ingredients without tossing. Sprinkle with cheese and artichoke hearts, if using. Cover and chill until ready to serve, then toss well, incorporating the lettuce into the dressing. Taste and add more dressing, if desired.

For pita plates, lay 1 whole round of bread on each plate and heap the salad on top.

Makes 4 servings.

Wheat Berry Salad

Wheat berries are whole-wheat kernels, hulled. You can't get any richer wheat goodness than this! You can find wheat berries in natural foods stores. It's best to soak them overnight before cooking, so plan ahead. Wheat berries double in volume during cooking.

    1 cup wheat berries
1¼ teaspoons salt
    1 cup chopped sweet onion, such as Vidalia, or
        scallions with their tops
    1 cucumber, peeled if waxed, diced
    4 large plum tomatoes, seeded and diced
    2 tablespoons extra-virgin olive oil
    2 tablespoons red wine vinegar
⅛ to ¼ teaspoon freshly ground black pepper
    1 tablespoon minced fresh basil or 1 teaspoon dried

Soak the wheat kernels in 1 quart water overnight. Drain. Cover with 1 quart of fresh water, add 1 teaspoon of the salt, and simmer in a saucepan until tender but still chewy, 40 to 50 minutes; drain.

When the wheat berries have cooled, mix them with the remaining ¼ teaspoon salt and remaining ingredients. Let stand at room temperature about 30 minutes before serving. Taste and add more oil or vinegar, if desired.

Makes 4 servings.

Asian Noodle Salad with Green Beans

Many of the Asian-inspired salads taste best when served at room temperature.

   Dressing (see below)
½ pound tender young green beans, cut diagonally into 2-inch lengths
12 ounces fresh Asian-style noodles or vermicelli
 6 scallions, cut diagonally into 1-inch pieces
 1 cup thinly sliced fennel or celery
 1 tablespoon sesame seeds, lightly toasted (page 298)

Dressing
 3 tablespoons canola oil
 1 teaspoon sesame oil
 3 tablespoons rice vinegar
 1 tablespoon naturally brewed soy sauce
 1 teaspoon sugar
 1 slice fresh ginger, finely minced
   A few dashes of hot pepper sauce

Prepare the dressing: Whisk together the canola oil, sesame oil, vinegar, soy sauce, sugar, ginger, and hot pepper sauce until the sugar is dissolved.

Cook the green beans in a large pot of boiling salted water until tender, about 5 minutes. Remove them with a slotted spoon and rinse them in cold water. Bring the water back to a rapid boil and cook the noodles until tender but not mushy, according to package directions. If there are no directions, start testing after 2 minutes. Drain and rinse the noodles in cold water.

Toss the noodles with the dressing in a large salad bowl. Add the green beans, scallions, and fennel and toss again. Sprinkle with sesame seeds.

Makes 4 servings.

Vegetable Antipasto

This light antipasto can be served before the pasta, as its name suggests, or as a luncheon dish. Serve with slices of crusty French bread.

¼ cup extra-virgin olive oil
2 tablespoons red wine vinegar
1 teaspoon chopped fresh oregano or ½ teaspoon dried
½ teaspoon salt
¼ teaspoon freshly ground pepper
2 cups cauliflowerets, cut into small pieces
1 small zucchini, sliced into ¼-inch-thick half-rounds
1 large carrot, pared and thinly sliced
1 small red onion, sliced and separated into rings
1 fennel bulb, cored and cut into 1-inch chunks (to prevent browning, do not cut until ready to mix with the dressing)
½ cup pitted ripe olives
1 pint cherry tomatoes
½ pound fresh whole-milk or part-skim mozzarella cheese (can be part-skim), diced
Romaine lettuce leaves

Combine the oil, vinegar, oregano, salt, and pepper in a deep bowl. Add the cauliflower, zucchini, carrot, onion, fennel, and olives. Toss well. Allow the vegetables to marinate at room temperature about 30 minutes, stirring occasionally. Cover and chill the vegetables.

When ready to serve, add the tomatoes and cheese and toss to combine. Line a platter with lettuce leaves and top with the vegetables.

Makes 6 servings.

Cannellini Bean and Tuna Salad

Italian tuna has a lovely taste, but it does come packed in olive oil. The cook can compensate, however, by draining off as much oil as possible and using very little additional oil in the salad.

2 (6- to 7-oz. each) cans Italian tuna *(tonno)*, drained and
   rinsed with wine vinegar
4 scallions, chopped
1 celery stalk with leaves, diced
1 tablespoon minced fresh flat-leaf parsley
1 tablespoon olive oil
2 to 3 tablespoons fresh lemon juice
⅛ to ¼ teaspoon freshly ground black pepper
2 cups cooked cannellini beans (page 328) or 1 (16-oz.) can
   cannellini beans (white kidney beans), drained and rinsed
8 large leaves chicory, torn into bite-size pieces

Combine the tuna, scallions, celery, parsley, oil, lemon juice, and pepper and toss to blend. Gently stir in the beans. Taste and add more lemon juice, if desired.

Divide the chicory among 4 salad plates. Heap the bean and tuna mixture on top.

Makes 4 servings.

Tomato, Tuna, and Bell Pepper Salad

A quick luncheon dish with lots of protein power.

2 large ripe tomatoes, seeded and diced
1 (7- to 7½-oz.) can water-packed white tuna, rinsed and flaked
1 green bell pepper, seeded and diced
1 celery stalk, diced
4 scallions with green tops, chopped
1 tablespoon chopped fresh flat-leaf parsley
2 tablespoons extra-virgin olive oil
1 to 2 tablespoons white wine vinegar
   Freshly ground black pepper
   Romaine lettuce leaves
   Large green Sicilian olives (optional), for garnish
   Crusty Italian rolls

Combine the tomatoes, tuna, bell pepper, celery, scallions, parsley, and oil in a medium bowl. Add vinegar and black pepper to taste, and allow the salad to marinate 15 minutes before serving.

Arrange lettuce on 2 or 3 salad plates. Heap the tuna mixture on top. Garnish with olives, if desired, and serve crusty rolls on the side.

Makes 2 or 3 servings.

Tuna and Cauliflower Salad

Simply rinsing tuna in cool water makes it much less salty.

  1 small head cauliflower
  1 tablespoon white vinegar
  1 (7- to 7½-oz.) can water-packed white tuna
  ¼ cup chopped sweet onion
10 to 12 stuffed green olives, sliced
  1 teaspoon drained capers
1½ tablespoons white wine vinegar
  1 teaspoon Dijon mustard
  ⅛ teaspoon freshly ground black pepper
  3 tablespoons olive oil

Trim off the leaves and core and separate the cauliflower into flowerets. Cut any extra-large flowerets in half. Cook the cauliflower with the vinegar in a pot of boiling salted water until crisp-tender, about 3 minutes. Drain and rinse in cold water.

Drain, rinse, and flake the tuna into a salad bowl. Add the onion, olives, and capers. Stir in the cauliflower.

Whisk together the vinegar, mustard, and pepper in a small bowl. Gradually whisk in the oil. Pour this vinaigrette over the salad and toss well. Cover and chill before serving.

Makes 4 servings.

Salmon, Peas, and Pasta Salad

A pretty main-dish salad for lunch or a quick supper. Cornichons are tiny, very sour pickles.

  1 cup nonfat plain yogurt
 ¼ cup mayonnaise
  1 tablespoon Dijon mustard
 ½ teaspoon white pepper
  1 tablespoon drained capers
  1 tablespoon chopped fresh dill or ½ teaspoon dried
  3 tablespoons finely chopped cornichons (optional)
  1 cup small pasta shells
1½ cups fresh shelled or frozen green peas
  1 (14½-oz.) can red salmon
  2 inner stalks of celery with leaves, chopped
 ¼ cup finely chopped red onion
     About 8 leaves of butter lettuce
  2 to 4 hard-cooked eggs (optional), peeled and sliced

Whisk together the yogurt, mayonnaise, mustard, and pepper in a salad bowl. Stir in the capers, dill, and cornichons, if using. Cook and drain the pasta; rinse until cool. Stir into the dressing.

Cook the peas in water to cover in a small saucepan until crisp-tender, about 3 minutes. Drain, cool, and stir into the pasta mixture.

Drain the salmon and break it into small chunks. Stir the salmon, celery, and red onion into the salad, cover, and chill until ready to serve.

Arrange butter lettuce on 4 plates, and divide the pasta salad among them. If desired, garnish with slices of hard-cooked egg.

Makes 4 servings.

Chicken Salad on the Light Side

This summer favorite is much quicker and easier to prepare if you start with boned breasts instead of the whole bird.

1½ pounds boneless, skinless chicken breasts
  1 quart Chicken-Mushroom Stock (page 333), canned broth, or prepared bouillon
  1 carrot, sliced
  1 onion, chopped
    A few pinches of dried herbs such as thyme and rosemary
 ½ cup mayonnaise
    About ½ cup nonfat plain yogurt
    White pepper
  2 Granny Smith apples, peeled, cored, and diced
  1 cup finely diced celery
 ½ cup dried cranberries, plumped in hot water and drained
 ½ cup pinc nuts, lightly toasted (page 298)
 ½ cup finely chopped fresh flat-leaf parsley
  1 bunch watercress, rinsed and tough stems removed
  1 pint cherry tomatoes, halved

Combine the chicken, stock, carrot, onion, and herbs in a large pot. Bring to a boil, reduce the heat, and simmer over low heat 10 to 15 min utes, until the chicken is just cooked through. Remove and chill the chicken. Save the broth for soup.

Mix the mayonnaise, yogurt, and white pepper to taste in a large bowl. Stir in the apples, celery, and cranberries. Dice the chicken and stir it into the dressing. Cover and chill.

When ready to serve, stir in the nuts and parsley. Add more yogurt, if desired. Mound the salad in the center of a platter and garnish with the watercress and cherry tomatoes.

Makes 6 servings.

Orange, Scallion, Radish, and Mint Salad

A refreshing salad with a Sicilian flavor.

4 navel oranges, peeled, white pith removed, and sliced into rounds
5 to 6 radishes, trimmed and thinly sliced
1 bunch scallions, cut diagonally into 1-inch lengths
3 tablespoons extra-virgin olive oil
  Salt and freshly ground black pepper
2 tablespoons finely chopped fresh mint
  Mint sprigs, for garnish

Arrange the orange rounds and radishes on a platter. Scatter the scallions on top. Drizzle with oil and season with salt and pepper to taste. Let stand at room temperature about 30 minutes before serving. Sprinkle with chopped mint and garnish with mint sprigs.

Makes 4 servings.

VARIATION

Orange, Cucumber, and Red Onion Salad

Substitute 1 peeled, sliced cucumber for the radishes and ¼ cup minced red onion for the scallions.

Spinach and Raspberry Salad

This simple and surprising combination relies on the tender quality of the spinach.

4 cups tender young spinach, stems removed,
     torn into bite-size pieces
4 cups bite-size pieces of leaf lettuce
¼ cup olive oil
     About 2 tablespoons raspberry vinegar
     Freshly ground black pepper
1 cup fresh raspberries

Combine greens in a salad bowl, cover, and chill. Just before serving, toss with oil, vinegar to taste, and pepper. Sprinkle with raspberries and serve.
Makes 4 servings.

Fennel and Grapefruit Salad

Perfect for serving with an oily fish, such as salmon or trout, this salad is light and refreshing.

2 large red or pink grapefruit
3 tablespoons olive oil
1 tablespoon chopped fresh mint or ½ teaspoon dried
¼ teaspoon salt
  Freshly ground black pepper
1 fennel bulb (about 1 lb.), trimmed and cored, and leaves reserved
  About ½ head romaine lettuce, washed, spun-dry, and
  torn into bite-size pieces

Remove the peel and white pith from the grapefruit. Working over a bowl to catch the juices, cut the grapefruit segments free of the encasing membrane, using a small serrated fruit knife. When no segments are left, squeeze the remaining membrane to release more juice.

Combine ⅓ cup of the grapefruit juice and 3 tablespoons olive oil in a salad bowl. Add the mint, salt, and pepper to taste. Cut the fennel into thin slices and stir it into the dressing. (Don't cut the fennel ahead of time, because it will turn brown.) Add the grapefruit segments and toss well.

Arrange the romaine lettuce on 4 salad plates. Top with the fennel-grapefruit mixture. Garnish with reserved fennel leaves.

Makes 4 servings.

New Wave Waldorf Salad

Chinese five-spice powder is found in supermarkets where Asian foods are sold, or you can make your own mix with equal amounts of ground anise, fennel seeds, cinnamon, cloves, and black pepper.

- 1 large seedless red grapefruit
- 2 Bosc or Bartlett pears
- 2 Rome apples
- 1 small bulb fennel, trimmed
- 3 tablespoons mayonnaise
- ¼ cup nonfat plain yogurt
- ½ teaspoon Chinese five-spice powder, or pinches of the five spices (see headnote)
- 1 cup seedless red grapes, halved
- ½ cup diced dried apricots
- 8 large leaves of Bibb lettuce

Remove the peel and white pith from the grapefruit. Working over a bowl to catch the juices, cut the grapefruit segments free of the encasing membrane, using a small serrated fruit knife. When no segments are left, squeeze the remaining membrane to release more juice.

Peel, core, and dice the pears, apples, and fennel, stirring them into the grapefruit juice as you work, to prevent browning.

Mix the mayonnaise and yogurt in another large bowl. Blend in the five-spice powder. With a slotted spoon, remove the pears, apples, and fennel from the grapefruit juice, draining them completely. Stir the pears, apples, fennel, grapefruit segments, grapes, and apricots into the dressing. Cover and chill until ready to serve. (The leftover grapefruit juice makes a refreshing beverage for the cook.)

Divide the lettuce leaves among 4 salad plates. Heap the fruit mixture on top.

Makes 4 servings.

Melon and Strawberry Fruit Salad with Yogurt

A tempting summer luncheon dish.

1 small cantaloupe, peeled, seeded, and cut into bite-size pieces
1 pint strawberries, hulled and halved lengthwise
1 cup seedless grapes
1 large banana, sliced
3 tablespoons honey, warmed
1 teaspoon vanilla extract
1 cup plain nonfat yogurt
   Butter lettuce leaves
½ cup chopped walnuts or ¼ cup chopped crystallized ginger (optional)

Combine and gently toss the fruits in a bowl. Whisk the honey and vanilla into the yogurt and blend it with the fruit. Line 6 individual salad bowls with lettuce leaves and divide the salad among them. Garnish with chopped nuts or chopped ginger, if desired. Serve immediately.

Makes 6 servings.

Never Give Up Desserts, Just Make Them Healthier

Beautiful, delicious, ripe fruits seem to have been designed by nature to be the pleasing conclusion to a good meal, and hidden in their sweet flesh is a powerhouse of antiaging compounds—vitamins, minerals, and phytochemicals. The problem is that many of us have become used to sugary, chocolatey, butter-filled, jam-packed, pastry-wrapped desserts, so placing before us, say, a perfectly ripe pear after dinner leaves us looking for a box of Oreos later. Sad but true.

But with just a little transformation, or culinary magic, fruits can be the basis of healthy desserts that have real appeal to the sweets-lover. For instance, poach that pear in a syrup or slice the fruit and bake it with a crisp nutty topping, and you'll have a dessert that will satisfy as well as contribute some real antioxidant and disease-fighting punch.

Apples and pears are rich in bone-building boron, plus soluble fiber. Bananas are loaded with potassium for the heart. Strawberries, melons, and raspberries are serious contributors of vitamin C. Cranberries and blueberries safeguard bladder health. Pineapple is high in manganese, another strong-bone mineral. And these are only the highlights. So how can we get ourselves and others to enjoy more fruits?

Besides trying some of the dessert recipes in this chapter, which do use many fruits, consider presentation when you serve fresh fruit as a dessert. If you and those you cook for don't reach for the fruit bowl after dinner, a simple matter of arranging the fruit on a plate may make a difference. For instance, peel and slice that ripe pear mentioned earlier, sprinkle it with a pinch of brown sugar, arrange it with a few pitted dates and one crisp gingersnap, and you'll have an attractive dessert that looks like a dessert. It's been my experience that people will eat more fresh fruit when it's attractively presented and requires no work.

Other nutritious components of desserts are cereals and grains, such as oats and wheat with their bonus of B vitamins; nuts, which are rich in vitamin E; dairy foods, which are high in calcium; and eggs, which, while not a superfood, are a great source of choline, a good memory food.

And desserts are fun, a little gift you give yourself when life is tough. Remember that *stressed* spelled backward is *desserts*.

Nectarine Mousse

*Smooth and sweet—you'd never know this mousse is a helping of vita-
mins A and C, plus calcium. I like the nutty crunch of amaretti (crisp
Italian almond cookies) as a topping.*

1 cup orange juice
2 envelopes unflavored gelatin
⅓ cup sugar
½ teaspoon natural almond flavoring
4 large ripe nectarines, peeled and chopped
1 cup nonfat plain yogurt
4 amaretti cookies (optional), crushed

Combine the juice, gelatin, and sugar in a small saucepan, stir, and let
stand 5 minutes. Warm the mixture over low heat, stirring, until the
gelatin and sugar are completely dissolved, 2 to 3 minutes. Stir in the
almond flavoring.

Puree the nectarines in a food processor. Blend in the gelatin mixture,
then the yogurt. Divide the mousse among 4 to 6 stemmed dessert dishes
or water goblets. Chill until set, several hours or overnight. Sprinkle
with amaretti crumbs, if desired.

Makes 4 to 6 servings.

Rosy Mulled Pears

Pears and wine are both sources of boron, a mineral that helps to keep bones strong.

1½ cups water
¾ cup sugar
1 cinnamon stick
1 vanilla bean
6 large Bartlett or Bosc pears, peeled, halved, and cored
½ cup dry red wine

Boil the water and sugar in a large saucepan, stirring, until all the sugar is dissolved. Add the cinnamon stick and vanilla bean. Use a slotted spoon to add the pear halves to the water. Add the wine, reduce heat, and gently simmer the pears, uncovered, until tender, 15 to 20 minutes, depending on ripeness. Remove the pears with a slotted spoon to a casserole dish with a cover.

Remove the cinnamon stick and vanilla bean. (They can be rinsed, dried, and used again.) Boil the syrup over medium-high heat until it's reduced to about 1½ cups. Cool it slightly, and pour it over the pears. Cover and chill the pears before serving.

Makes 6 servings.

Maple-Walnut Bananas

A very special dessert that you can whip up in 10 minutes, with the happy knowledge that bananas and walnuts are heart-healthy foods and that even nonfat frozen yogurt is adding calcium to your diet.

¼ cup maple syrup
⅓ cup unsalted walnut halves or pieces
 1 teaspoon unsalted butter
 3 medium bananas, sliced crosswise
 4 scoops nonfat frozen butterscotch or vanilla yogurt

Stir the syrup, walnuts, and butter together in a medium skillet over low heat until the butter has melted. Add the bananas and barely simmer 5 minutes, stirring often. Divide the bananas among 4 dessert dishes and top with the frozen yogurt.

Makes 4 servings.

Figs Poached with Candied Ginger

This light, flavorful dessert is a real pick-me-up for the immune system—both ginger and figs are rich sources of phytochemicals. Crystallized (or candied) ginger is found in some natural foods and specialty stores, and it's worth the hunt. Calimyrna dried figs are large, soft, and golden in color.

1　(8-oz.) package Calimyrna dried figs
6　slices crystallized ginger, halved
　　Apple juice

Combine the figs and ginger in a saucepan. Add just enough apple juice to barely cover them, and bring mixture to a boil. Reduce the heat so that the juice is simmering, and cook the figs, uncovered, 20 minutes, stirring often.

Cool slightly, then pour into a serving bowl, cover, and chill the figs in their juice.

Makes 20 to 24 figs, about 6 servings.

Blueberry-Raspberry Summer Pudding

Summer pudding, a favorite in Great Britain, should be an easy, lazy dessert, so I'm not suggesting that you sieve the fruit to remove seeds and skins (which, after all, are high in fiber). The pudding is perfectly delicious this way, using the whole fruit.

 5 cups fresh or frozen blueberries
 ½ cup water
 ⅔ cup plus 2 tablespoons sugar
 ½ teaspoon ground cinnamon
 ¼ teaspoon ground nutmeg
 6 slices firm white sandwich bread, crusts removed
    About ¼ cup applesauce
 1 pint fresh raspberries
    Nonfat frozen vanilla yogurt (optional)

Combine the blueberries, water, ⅔ cup sugar, cinnamon, and nutmeg in a large saucepan over medium heat. Bring the mixture to a boil, reduce the heat, and simmer, stirring often, about 15 minutes, until the fruit is slightly thickened. Cool.

Cut the bread slices in half and spread them with a thin layer of applesauce. Line a loaf pan with plastic wrap. Arrange 4 halves, applesauce side down, in the pan. Spread ⅓ of the blueberry sauce over the bread. Repeat layers twice more. Cover with plastic wrap and chill overnight.

Mix the raspberries with remaining 2 tablespoons sugar, stir, and chill about 2 hours, stirring occasionally.

Carefully invert the pudding onto a serving dish, removing all plastic wrap. Top with raspberries. If desired, serve with frozen yogurt as a topping.

Makes 6 servings.

Triple-Ginger Yogurt

If you love the spicy hot taste of ginger, you'll enjoy this dessert.

2½ cups nonfat plain yogurt (without gelatin or other stabilizers)
 ¼ cup packed light brown sugar
 ¼ cup ginger marmalade
 1 tablespoon finely chopped crystallized ginger
 4 gingersnaps, crushed

Place a paper coffee filter in a strainer, add the yogurt, and drain over a bowl, in the refrigerator, 1 hour. Discard the liquid in the bowl. Whisk the brown sugar into the slightly thickened yogurt; stir in the marmalade and chopped ginger. Divide the yogurt among 4 stemmed dessert dishes, cover, and chill.

Just before serving, sprinkle the desserts with gingersnap crumbs.
Makes 4 servings.

Minted Melon and Grapes with Yogurt

This is a late-summer dessert, when local melons are ripe and the first grapes have come into the market. Fresh *mint is a necessity for this dish.*

1   small ripe cantaloupe, peeled, seeded, and cut into bite-size
    chunks, or 2 (16-oz.) packages frozen melon balls, thawed and
    drained
2   cups seedless green grapes
    About 3 tablespoons honey
1   tablespoon minced fresh mint
1   cup nonfat plain yogurt
    About 1 tablespoon dark brown sugar
    Mint sprigs, for garnish (optional)

Combine the cantaloupe and grapes in a serving bowl. Warm the honey just enough to make it thin and pourable. A few seconds in the microwave will do it. Whisk the honey and mint into the yogurt. Taste the yogurt, adding more honey, if desired. Stir the yogurt into the fruit.

Divide the fruit among 6 dessert dishes. Sprinkle a little brown sugar on top. Garnish with mint sprigs, if desired. Serve immediately.

Makes 6 servings

Strawberry Sundaes with Balsamic Vinegar

A "grown-up" sundae, light and elegant. The balsamic vinegar adds a rich undercurrent of flavor without tasting "vinegary." Amaretti are crisp Italian almond cookies.

     1   quart ripe strawberries, rinsed and hulled
     3   tablespoons balsamic vinegar
    ¼   cup sugar
    ⅓   cup orange juice
    1½   pints (3 cups) nonfat frozen strawberry yogurt
     6   amaretti cookies, crushed
    ⅓   cups slivered almonds, toasted (see Note below)

Slice the strawberries into a bowl, add the vinegar, and lightly toss them together. Allow them to marinate 10 minutes. Stir the sugar into the orange juice until dissolved, and add syrup to the strawberries. Toss again and refrigerate at least 1 hour, stirring once or twice.

To assemble, arrange scoops of frozen yogurt in 6 dessert dishes. Top with the marinated strawberries. Sprinkle with the amaretti crumbs and toasted almonds.

Makes 6 servings.

NOTE

To toast almonds or other nuts and seeds, place them in a small, dry nonstick skillet over medium heat. Toast, stirring constantly, 3 to 5 minutes, until they are golden. Immediately remove them from the pan and cool.

Cranberry-apple Bread Pudding

Vitamin C, B vitamins, calcium, iron, boron, and fiber in one old-fashioned, comforting dessert.

3 large eggs
⅔ cup sugar
¼ teaspoon ground cinnamon
¼ teaspoon ground nutmeg, plus more for sprinkling
⅛ teaspoon salt
2 cups whole or low-fat milk
1 teaspoon vanilla extract
2 cups diced, crustless whole-wheat bread
1 large apple, peeled, cored, and chopped into small pieces
½ cup coarsely chopped fresh or frozen cranberries
¼ cup golden raisins

Butter a 2½-quart glass casserole dish (preferably shallow rather than deep). Whip the eggs with a whisk until light. Blend in the sugar, spices, and salt. Whisk in the milk and vanilla.

Add the bread to prepared casserole dish. Mix the apple, cranberries, and raisins with the bread. Pour the egg mixture over all, pressing the bread down. Sprinkle the top with additional nutmeg. Let stand 15 minutes. Set casserole dish in a larger baking pan.

Preheat the oven to 350F (175C). Place the baking dishes in the oven on the middle shelf and pour hot water into the outer pan. Bake 40 to 45 minutes or until set in the center. Serve warm or at room temperature.

Makes 6 servings.

Apricot and Pear Clafouti

A clafouti is an easily assembled French baked dessert that's a cross between a big pancake and a flan. It's essential that the pears be ripe and soft, or use canned pears.

1¼ cups whole or low-fat milk
⅔ cup unbleached all-purpose flour
 2 large eggs
 1 large egg white
⅓ cup granulated sugar
 1 teaspoon vanilla extract
½ teaspoon ground ginger
⅛ teaspoon salt
½ tablespoon butter
1¼ cups peeled, diced ripe pear (2 pears)
¾ cup dried apricots, snipped into pieces with a kitchen shears
   Powdered sugar, for garnish

Preheat the oven to 350F (175C).

Whisk together the milk, flour, eggs, egg white, sugar, vanilla, ginger, and salt in a bowl or process in a blender or food processor.

Melt the butter in a 10-inch cast-iron skillet or any heavy skillet with a flameproof handle over very low heat. Pour in ½ cup of the batter and cook until it sets, like a crêpe, 3 to 5 minutes. Scatter the diced pears over the cooked layer, followed by the apricots. Pour the remaining batter over all.

Bake on the middle shelf until the clafouti is set, puffed, and golden, about 50 minutes. It will fall a little. Sprinkle with powdered sugar and serve at once, cut into wedges.

Makes 6 servings.

Blueberry Cobbler with Cornmeal-Buttermilk Topping

An old-fashioned dessert that's still an easy favorite. Blueberries contain phytochemicals that help to prevent bladder infections and fight other bacteria as well.

3½ cups fresh blueberries
½ cup sugar
2 tablespoons instant flour, such as Wondra
¼ teaspoon ground cinnamon

Topping
1 cup unbleached all-purpose flour
½ cup cornmeal, preferably whole grain
¼ cup granulated sugar
1 teaspoon baking powder
½ teaspoon baking soda
¼ teaspoon ground cinnamon
1 large egg, beaten
½ cup buttermilk or sour milk (page 338)
3 tablespoons vegetable oil

Preheat the oven to 375F (190C).

Put the blueberries in a 9-inch glass pie pan or a 9-inch-square ceramic baking dish. Mix together the sugar, flour, and cinnamon, and stir it into the blueberries.

Prepare the topping: Sift together the flour, cornmeal, sugar, baking powder, soda, and cinnamon into a medium bowl. Whisk together the egg, buttermilk, and oil. Stir the liquid ingredients into the dry ingredients until just blended. Spoon the batter over the fruit, and spread it to the edges of the pan.

Bake in the top third of the oven about 25 minutes, until the top is golden brown, the topping is cooked through, and the filling is bubbly throughout. If the top browns too fast, lay a sheet of foil over it. Cool until just warm and serve.

Makes 6 servings.

Blueberry-Banana Shortcakes

The shortcakes are made with oil and banana puree instead of butter and served with nonfat frozen yogurt rather than whipped cream for a low-fat version of an old favorite.

    Sauce (see below)
2 cups unbleached all-purpose flour
2 tablespoons sugar
1 tablespoon baking powder
½ teaspoon salt
¼ teaspoon ground nutmeg
¼ teaspoon ground ginger
¾ cup banana puree (1 ripe banana)
¼ cup vegetable oil
    Nonfat frozen vanilla yogurt

Sauce
6 cups fresh or frozen blueberries
¾ cup sugar
1 teaspoon ground cinnamon
¾ cup water

Prepare the sauce: Combine the sauce ingredients in a medium saucepan and bring to a boil, stirring often. Reduce heat and simmer 8 minutes or until thick but pourable, stirring occasionally. Cool completely. Makes 3 cups of sauce.

Preheat the oven to 400F (205C). Sift together the flour, sugar, baking powder, salt, nutmeg, and ginger.

Whisk the banana puree and oil together with a fork, and stir banana mixture into the dry ingredients to make a soft dough. (If it doesn't hold together, stir in 1 or 2 teaspoons of milk.)

On a floured board, form the dough into 6 biscuits. Place them on an ungreased baking sheet and bake on the top rack until golden, 12 to 15 minutes. Cool until they're just warm, or rewarm when ready to serve.

To serve, split the shortcakes and divide them among 6 dessert dishes. Top with the sauce and dollops of frozen yogurt.

Makes 6 servings.

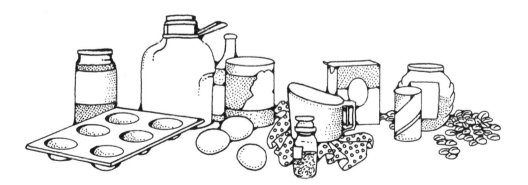

Fall Fruits Crisp

Make this warm dessert, perfect for the cool days of autumn, when the first fresh cranberries are available.

Topping (see below)
¾ cup sugar
¾ cup chopped fresh or frozen cranberries
2 to 3 cooking apples
2 ripe pears

Topping
½ cup packed dark brown sugar
½ cup unbleached all-purpose flour
½ teaspoon ground cinnamon
½ teaspoon ground ginger
¼ teaspoon ground nutmeg
Pinch of salt
¼ cup (½ stick) unsalted butter, chilled
½ cup uncooked regular or quick-cooking oatmeal
½ cup pecans

Preheat the oven to 375F (190C).

Prepare the topping: Mix together the brown sugar, flour, spices, and salt in a food processor. Cut in the butter until the mixture resembles coarse meal. Add the oats and pecans. Process briefly until the pecans are coarsely chopped. Alternatively, the pecans can be chopped by hand, the topping mixed in a bowl, and the butter cut in with a pastry cutter. Set the topping aside.

Mix together the sugar and cranberries in a 12-inch glass pie pan. Peel and thinly slice enough apples and pears to fill the pan, tossing them with the sugar occasionally to prevent browning. When the pan is full, press the fruit down into an even layer. Sprinkle the topping over all and press that into a layer.

Bake on the middle shelf 50 minutes or until the fruit is tender and the topping nicely browned. If the topping browns before the fruit is cooked, cover it loosely with a sheet of foil. Serve warm from the pan.

Makes 6 to 8 servings.

Crustless Ricotta Pie with Wheat Berries

Dispensing with the pastry shell makes this a low-fat version of the traditional Italian Easter pie, pizza dolce, *made with wheat berries or rice. You can't get better whole-grain goodness than wheat berries, rich in B vitamins and vitamin E.*

½ cup uncooked whole-wheat kernels (available in natural foods stores)
1 tablespoon plain dry bread crumbs
1½ pounds whole-milk ricotta cheese, drained
3 large eggs
½ cup sugar
⅛ teaspoon salt
1 teaspoon vanilla extract
¼ teaspoon grated lemon peel
2 tablespoons candied chopped lemon peel
2 tablespoons candied chopped citron

Soak the wheat kernels in water overnight. Drain, cover with fresh water, and simmer until tender, 40 to 50 minutes. Drain. (If you cook more than you need, extras can be frozen for later use, such as Wheat Berry Salad, page 276.) Measure 1 cup cooked wheat to use in the pie.

Preheat the oven to 325F (165C). Butter a 10-inch glass pie pan or quiche dish. Scatter bread crumbs over the bottom and sides.

Whip the ricotta until creamy and smooth in a food processor or by hand with a heavy whisk. Blend in the eggs, sugar, salt, vanilla, and lemon peel. Stir in the candied fruits and wheat kernels. Spoon the mixture into the prepared pan. Bake until the cake is set 1 inch from the center, 45 to 50 minutes. Cool completely before cutting.

Makes 8 servings.

VARIATIONS

For a crowd, I sometimes double this recipe and bake it in a 13 × 9-inch pan, then serve it cut into squares with a fresh fruit accompaniment, such as sugared strawberries or raspberries.

Maple-Walnut Carrot Cake

A dessert rich with ingredients that are actually good for you, such as carrots (beta-carotene), walnuts (B vitamins), raisins (iron) and yogurt (calcium). And there's no need to frost this moist, flavorful cake!

2 cups unbleached all-purpose flour
2 teaspoons baking soda
½ teaspoon baking powder
½ teaspoon salt
1 teaspoon ground cinnamon
3 large eggs, beaten (see Note below)
1 cup nonfat plain yogurt
½ cup sugar
½ cup maple syrup
½ cup vegetable oil
1 teaspoon natural maple flavoring
3 cups loosely packed grated carrots (6 to 8)
1½ cups chopped walnuts
1 cup golden raisins

Preheat the oven to 350F (175C). Spray a 13 × 9-inch baking pan with nonstick cooking spray or butter and flour it.

Sift together the flour, soda, baking powder, salt, and cinnamon into a large bowl. Beat together the eggs, yogurt, sugar, syrup, oil, and maple flavoring in a bowl or use a food processor. Combine the carrots, nuts, and raisins in another bowl.

Pour the liquid ingredients into the dry ingredients, and beat until blended. Fold in the carrot mixture. Spoon the batter into the prepared pan.

Bake on the middle rack until a wooden pick or cake tester inserted in the center comes out clean, 30 to 35 minutes. If the top browns too quickly, lay a sheet of foil over it. Cool in the pan on a wire rack. Cut into squares to serve.

Makes 16 to 20 servings.

NOTE
If preferred, use 1 egg and ½ cup egg substitute for the 3 eggs.

Oatmeal-Apricot Morsels

A soft cookie with great grain goodness and the powerhouse of vitamin A in apricots. Much better for you than store-bought "fat-free" cookies, whose first ingredient is sugar.

1½ cups unbleached all-purpose flour
 1 teaspoon baking powder
 ½ teaspoon ground cinnamon
 ½ teaspoon salt
1¾ cups uncooked quick-cooking or regular oatmeal
 1 cup loosely packed diced dried apricots
 ½ cup canola oil
 2 large eggs or ½ cup egg substitute
 1 cup packed dark brown sugar
 1 teaspoon vanilla extract
 ¼ cup orange juice

Preheat the oven to 350F (175C).

Sift together the flour, baking powder, cinnamon, and salt into a medium bowl. Mix together the oats and apricots in another bowl. With an electric mixer or by hand, beat the eggs, oil, brown sugar, and vanilla until well blended. Beat in the orange juice, then the flour mixture. Remove from the mixer, if using, and stir in the oats and apricots by hand.

Drop the batter by heaping teaspoons, spaced 1 inch apart onto a non-stick baking sheet, and bake until golden, 10 to 11 minutes. Continue baking in batches until all the batter has been used. Cool completely on wire racks.

Makes about 4 dozen cookies.

Chocolate-Almond Torte with Peaches

This is a lighter-than-usual torte, but still dark and delicious. Peaches provide a refreshing counterpoint.

    Peach Topping (see below)
1¼ cups unbleached all-purpose flour
 ¼ cup cornstarch
1¼ teaspoons baking soda
 ¼ teaspoon salt
 ½ cup unsweetened cocoa powder
 ¾ cup granulated sugar
 1 cup water
 1 teaspoon vanilla extract
 ½ teaspoon natural almond flavoring
 ⅓ cup canola oil
 1 large whole egg
 1 large egg white
 ¼ cup slivered almonds
    Confectioner's sugar

Peach Topping

 4 large ripe fresh peaches, peeled and sliced, or
    2 (15-oz.) cans cling peach slices in fruit juice, drained
 ½ teaspoon natural almond flavoring
 1 tablespoon fresh lemon juice (optional)
 2 tablespoons sugar

Prepare the topping: Mix the peaches with the almond flavoring and lemon juice. Toss fresh peaches with the sugar; if using canned peaches, omit sugar. Cover and refrigerate peaches until needed.

Heat the oven to 325F (165C). Spray a 9-inch-round cake pan with nonstick cooking spray. Line the bottom with wax paper and spray the paper as well.

Sift together the flour, cornstarch, soda, and salt into a bowl; set aside.

Stir together the cocoa and granulated sugar in a large bowl. Beat in the water, vanilla, and almond flavoring, then the oil, and finally the egg and egg white, beating them in thoroughly. Beat in the flour mixture until smooth. Pour into the prepared pan.

Gently sprinkle the almonds as evenly as possible on the batter. They will sink a bit but will remain on top of the torte. Bake the torte on the middle rack 45 to 50 minutes or until a wooden pick or cake tester inserted in the center comes out clean. Cool in the pan on a wire rack 10 minutes.

Remove the torte from the pan, peel off the wax paper, and turn the cake upright; cool completely on a wire rack. Place cooled cake on a serving plate and sprinkle it with powdered sugar.

To serve, cut into wedges. Place the wedges on dessert plates and spoon peaches on the side.

Makes 8 servings.

Beverages—A Toast to the Good Life

❧❧

Beverages can be another source of protective vitamins, minerals, and phytochemicals. In recent research, tea has come to the forefront as a defender against cancer. The world's most popular beverage is rich in polyphenols, potent compounds that reduce the risk of developing tumors. Only nonherbal teas—black, green, or oolong—contain polyphenols.

Herbal teas, however, have their own special properties. Ginseng tea has been esteemed in Asia for thousands of years as a stimulant and prolonger of life. Ginger tea (and ginger ale that is made with real ginger, not artificial flavor) is a digestive aid, a nausea remedy, and a possible treatment for arthritis. Rose hips tea is bursting with antioxidant vitamin C, just the hot tonic to help ease symptoms of the common cold. Mint is a digestive aid and may also be a decongestant; herbal folklore credits this fragrant herb with promoting cheerfulness.

Strained fruit and vegetable juices are generally rich in antioxidant vitamins but don't contain all the goodness of the whole-plant product, such as flavonoids (in citrus membranes) and fiber. Unstrained juice drinks, however, such as those you might whip up in a food processor or blender, lose nothing in the processing. Such a juice drink can be an appetizing morning beverage for those who are feeling too rushed and stressed for solid food.

Red wine has been getting its share of attention recently as a heart

311

protector and defender against cancer. Two phytochemicals in red wine, resveratrol and quercetin, have been found to inhibit blood clotting and improve cholesterol levels. Quercetin is also a potent anticancer chemical. Red grape juice shares in these beneficial compounds.

With moderate activity, we have to replace two to three quarts of water every day. Juices in general can contribute to one's overall water intake. (Tea and coffee are not considered good substitutes for water, because they are diuretics.) Sometimes we stop being thirsty before our body's needs are met, so if you're concerned about hydration, juices can help.

Water is the ultimate beverage. It's involved in every body process. It fights fatigue. It cools menopausal hot flashes and helps the body to maintain an even temperature. And it helps to cleanse the skin and keep it soft and pliable. Whatever other beverages you enjoy, be sure to include plenty of good plain water every day.

A toast to your very good health!

Hot Ginger Tea for Two

Just the beverage to brew at home after consuming a heavy meal else-where. Ginger calms the stomach and relieves intestinal distress.

 2 teaspoons loose oolong tea
 1 teaspoon honey
 ½ teaspoon ground ginger
    About 2 cups boiling water
 2 thin slices of lemon (optional)

Pour a little boiling water into a 3-cup teapot to heat the pot before making the tea; drain.

Add the tea leaves, honey, and ginger to the pot. Add 2 cups boiling water or a little more if you prefer a weaker brew. Stir once and allow the tea to steep 3 to 5 minutes.

To serve, pour through a tea strainer into 2 cups. If desired, add lemon slices.

Makes 2 cups.

Iced Green Tea with Ginger

Polyphenols and catechins, chemical compounds found in green tea, oolong tea, and, to a lesser extent, in black tea, help clean up damaging free radicals in the body.

For longer storage of ginger, peeled slices can be wrapped in plastic wrap and frozen. They will thaw in minutes at room temperature. Another storage method is to place the slices in a small jar with enough dry white wine or dry vermouth to cover; refrigerate. Fresh ginger will keep for months by either method.

3 to 4 slices fresh ginger
3 tablespoons honey
1 quart (4 cups) boiling water
4 teaspoons loose green tea or 4 tea bags
    Ice cubes

Pour a little boiling water into a 4-cup teapot to heat the pot before making the tea. Drain.

Put the ginger and honey in the pot, and add about ½ cup of the boiling water. Let stand for a few minutes. Stir to dissolve the honey, and press the ginger with the back of a spoon to release its flavor.

Add the green tea and the remaining 3½ cups boiling water. Steep the tea about 20 minutes, then pour through a strainer into a large pitcher. When ready to serve, add ice to the pitcher, or pour the tea over ice in tall glasses.

Makes 4 servings.

Cheery After-Dinner-Mint Tea

Herbal folklore credits mint with being a cheer-up herb that brightens the spirits in times of stress. Modern herbalists note that mint is an aid to digestion, relieving a whole range of tummy miseries—a fact that accounts for the peppermint taste of many over-the-counter antacids. In addition, black tea contains astringent tannins, which help to relieve diarrhea.

1 tablespoon chopped fresh mint
2 teaspoons loose black tea (such as Darjeeling), or 2 tea bags
3 cups boiling water
   Raw sugar (optional)

Pour a little boiling water into a 3-cup teapot to heat the pot before making the tea; drain.

Put the mint and tea in the pot. Add the 3 cups of boiling water. Allow the tea to steep 3 to 5 minutes before serving. Pass the sugar, if desired.

Makes 3 cups

Mulled Grape Juice

A heartwarming beverage for a chilly evening. Red grapes are rich in resveratrol and quercetin, phytochemicals that protect against heart disease and cancer.

      Juice of 1 lemon
  2   cups water
  2   cinnamon sticks
  8   whole cloves
  1   quart red grape juice

   Combine the lemon juice, water, cinnamon stick, and cloves in a saucepan and slowly bring them to a boil. Add the grape juice and heat until hot but not boiling. Strain into a heatproof pitcher. Serve hot in small cups.
   Makes 6 servings.

Pineapple-Ginger Punch

This refreshing punch is rich in boron, a great bone builder.

      Ice cubes
  1   cup pineapple juice
      About 1 cup ginger ale
      Mint sprigs

   Fill 2 (12-oz.) glasses with ice cubes. Divide the pineapple juice between the glasses. Top with the ginger ale. Garnish with mint sprigs and serve immediately.
   Makes 2 servings.

Tropical Smoothie

Here's an antioxidant pick-me-up that's tastier than most nutrition-supplement drinks.

1 very ripe medium mango, peeled and diced
1 banana, sliced
1 cup orange juice
1 cup pineapple juice
1 tablespoon fresh lime juice
1 tablespoon honey
4 ice cubes
   Lime slices, for garnish (optional)

   Combine all ingredients except lime slices in a blender and puree until smooth. Pour into chilled glasses and serve. If desired, garnish each glass with a lime slice.
   Makes 4 cups, 3 or 4 servings.

Banana and Orange Frappé

Can't stomach solid food in the morning? Try this sweet solution. Bananas are great stomach soothers.

1 large ripe banana, cut into chunks
1 cup orange juice
1 tablespoon honey
½ cup nonfat plain yogurt

   Combine all the ingredients in a blender and blend until smooth and frothy. Pour into 2 glasses and serve immediately.
   Makes 2 servings.

Basic Recipes with Many Uses

The recipes in the following section are for foods that are useful in preparing many different dishes, such as a variety of tomato sauces for every purpose. Some of these recipes produce foods that can be used both as component ingredients and as finished dishes, such as Cannellini Beans, and some are condiments: Cinnamon Sugar or Spicy Pepper Mix.

In today's home kitchens, we don't usually have the abundance of meaty bones and vegetable parings that restaurant chefs can use to simmer for hours in 40-quart stockpots. My soup stock recipes, therefore, call for less cooking time and for chicken that doesn't have to be discarded after the stock is made. But if you happen to have a leftover roast chicken or turkey carcass that hasn't been picked too clean, it too makes a lovely stock. Simply add many of the same flavoring ingredients, add enough water to come about an inch above the bones, and simmer for an hour or so. Strain, cool, and freeze. What a bonus!

319

Italian Tomato Sauce with Mushrooms
(Salsa di Pomodoro e Funghi)

Two kinds of mushrooms give this sauce an intense, earthy flavor.

½ ounce dried porcini mushrooms
1 cup hot water
3 tablespoons olive oil
8 ounces fresh brown mushrooms, cleaned and sliced
1 to 2 garlic cloves, minced
1 (28-oz.) can imported Italian plum tomatoes with puree
½ teaspoon salt
¼ teaspoon freshly ground black pepper
1 tablespoon chopped fresh basil or ½ teaspoon dried
1 tablespoon chopped fresh flat-leaf parsley

Soak the dried mushrooms in the hot water for about a half hour. Drain, reserving the liquid. Rinse each mushroom carefully under cool running water. Chop the porcini and set aside. Arrange a paper coffee filter in a fine-meshed strainer and strain the soaking liquid; reserve.

Heat 2 tablespoons of the oil in a nonstick 10-inch skillet, and sauté the fresh mushrooms over medium-high heat, stirring often, until they release their juices and begin to brown.

Reduce the heat to low, add the remaining tablespoon of oil, and sauté the garlic for 1 minute. It should not brown.

Add the porcini, their soaking liquid, tomatoes, salt, and pepper. (If using dried basil, add it with the salt and pepper.) Cook over medium heat, uncovered, stirring often, for about 30 minutes, until reduced to the desired sauce consistency. Stir in the fresh basil and parsley.

Makes 2½ to 3 cups, enough for 1 pound of pasta.

Italian Marinara Sauce

Marinara *means "of the sea." Even so, it's not a fish sauce—although it may be enriched with anchovies—but a spicy, garlicky herb sauce from the south of Italy. This recipe yields enough for 1 pound of thin linguine or thin spaghetti, lightly sauced.*

3 tablespoons olive oil
2 Italian frying peppers (green), seeded and finely diced
1 to 2 dried hot red chiles
2 to 3 garlic cloves, finely chopped
1 (28-oz.) can imported Italian plum tomatoes with puree
4 anchovy fillets, chopped (optional)
¼ teaspoon salt, or ¾ teaspoon if omitting anchovies
¼ teaspoon freshly ground black pepper
1 tablespoon chopped fresh oregano or ½ teaspoon dried
1 tablespoon chopped fresh basil or ½ teaspoon dried
1 tablespoon chopped fresh flat leaf parsley

Heat the oil in a 10-inch skillet and sauté the frying pepper over medium heat, stirring often, until lightly colored, 3 to 5 minutes. Reduce the heat to low, add the chile and garlic, and continue to sauté for 1 minute, or until the garlic is yellow but not brown.

Add the tomatoes, anchovies if you wish, salt, and pepper. (If using dried herbs, add them with the salt and pepper.) Cook over medium heat, uncovered, stirring often, for about 30 minutes, until reduced to the desired sauce consistency. Stir in the fresh oregano, basil, and parsley. Remove the chile before using.

Makes 2½ cups.

Spanish Tomato Sauce with Olives

A savory sauce with chunky vegetables that can really enliven any plainly cooked chicken.

    3   tablespoons olive oil
    1   large red bell pepper, seeded and sliced into strips
    1   large yellow onion, sliced into half-rounds
    2   garlic cloves, finely chopped
    1   (28-oz.) can imported Italian plum tomatoes with puree
    2   tablespoons tomato paste
    ½   teaspoon dried basil
    ¼   teaspoon salt
    ¼   teaspoon freshly ground black pepper
    ½   cup ripe olives, halved
    ½   cup stuffed green olives, halved
    1   tablespoon chopped fresh cilantro or flat-leaf parsley

Heat the oil in a 10-inch skillet and sauté the bell pepper and onion over medium heat, stirring often, until lightly colored, 3 to 5 minutes. Reduce the heat to low, add the garlic, and continue to sauté for 1 minute, or until the garlic is yellow but not brown.

Chop the tomatoes. Add the tomatoes, tomato paste, basil, salt, and pepper to the skillet. Cook over low heat, with cover ajar, stirring often, for 20 to 25 minutes, until reduced to the desired sauce consistency. Stir in the cilantro or parsley.

Makes 3 cups.

French Tomato Sauce

Herbes de Provence, butter, and lots of shallots give this sauce its French flavor. An excellent dressing for plain fish.

1 (28-oz.) can imported Italian plum tomatoes with puree
1 tablespoon olive oil
2 tablespoons unsalted butter
½ cup chopped shallots
½ teaspoon salt
¼ teaspoon freshly ground black pepper
1 teaspoon chopped fresh thyme or ⅛ teaspoon dried
1 teaspoon chopped fresh rosemary or ⅛ teaspoon dried
1 teaspoon chopped fresh tarragon or summer savory or
    ⅛ teaspoon dried
1 tablespoon chopped fresh flat-leaf parsley

Put the tomatoes through a food mill to remove the seeds. Alternatively, remove the tomatoes from the puree with a slotted spoon, cut each in half, and remove the seeds, then chop the tomatoes into a small dice. Return the puree to the seeded tomatoes.

Heat the oil and butter in a 10-inch skillet and sauté the shallots over medium heat, stirring often, until lightly colored, 3 to 5 minutes.

Add the tomatoes, salt, and pepper. (If using dried herbs, add them with the salt and pepper.) Cook over medium heat, uncovered, stirring often, for about 30 minutes, until reduced to the desired sauce consistency. Stir in the fresh thyme, rosemary, tarragon, and parsley.

Makes about 2½ cups.

Baked Tomato Sauce

This tomato sauce achieves a deep, rich flavor without the addition of any meat. It requires very little stirring, and it's no trouble at all to make a large batch at one time. (But if you double the recipe, use two pans.) A single recipe makes enough sauce for 2 pounds of pasta.

¼ cup olive oil
2 garlic cloves, finely chopped
1 large red bell pepper, seeded and diced
1 large green bell pepper, seeded and diced
1 dried hot red chile
2 (28-oz.) cans imported Italian plum tomatoes in puree
½ to 1 teaspoon dried oregano (Oregano imparts a
   "pizza" flavor; use it to your taste.)
1 teaspoon salt
½ teaspoon black pepper
1 tablespoon Basil Pesto (page 327) or finely minced fresh basil
1 tablespoon finely minced fresh flat-leaf parsley

Preheat the oven to 375F (190C). Coat the bottom of a large (13 × 9-inch) nonreactive baking pan with the oil. Scatter the garlic, bell peppers, and chile in the pan, and bake on the middle rack until sizzling but without browning the garlic, about 10 minutes.

Remove the pan from the oven. Add the tomatoes, oregano, salt, and pepper; stir well. Make a mental note of the level of sauce in the pan. Bake until reduced to two-thirds of its original volume, about 50 minutes. Stir once during the cooking process.

Remove the chile. Stir in the pesto or basil and the parsley. Bake 5 minutes longer.

Makes 5½ to 6 cups.

VARIATION

For a kind of "Italian sausage" flavor without the fat, stir in ½ teaspoon crushed fennel seeds with the oregano. Add extra freshly ground black pepper when the sauce is finished. Fennel and pepper are the distinctive flavors of Italian sausage.

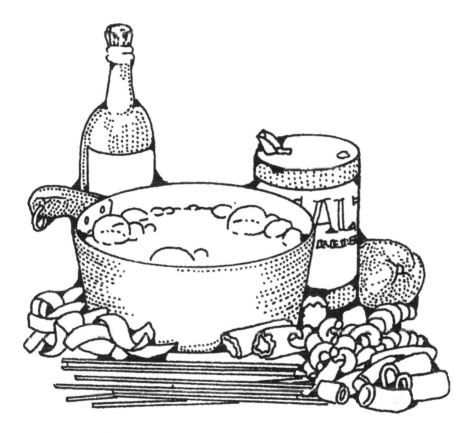

Make-It-Easy Polenta

A hearty pasta substitute—the Mediterranean's answer to our cornmeal mush. If you have a large double boiler, you won't have to stir this polenta for a half hour as called for in many traditional recipes.

- 1 cup cold water
- 1 cup polenta (coarsely ground cornmeal, preferably whole-grain)
- 3 cups Chicken-Mushroom Stock (page 333), Vegetable Stock (page 331), canned broth, or prepared bouillon
- ¼ cup freshly grated Parmesan cheese
- ½ teaspoon salt (optional)
- Freshly ground black pepper

Blend the water and polenta in a 2-cup (or larger) measuring pitcher. Pour the stock into the top of the double boiler and bring it to a boil over direct heat. Gradually add the polenta mixture, stirring with a whisk to prevent clumping. Lower the heat and continue stirring until the polenta thickens, about 30 minutes. (Be careful: Boiling polenta can splatter quite high. Keep heat low, and be ready to move the pan off-heat if necessary.)

Meanwhile, bring 2 inches of water to a boil in the bottom of the double boiler. Put the top of the double boiler containing the thickened polenta in place. Cook with cover slightly ajar for 45 minutes. Thoroughly whisk every 15 minutes to smooth any lumps.

Whisk in cheese, salt, if using, and pepper to your taste. Use immediately, serving heaping spoonfuls of polenta with the topping of your choice

Makes about 3½ cups.

VARIATION

Chill the polenta in an oiled 11 × 7-inch pan and cool. Cut into squares before reheating.

Basil Pesto

Make this in the summer when fresh basil is plentiful. Freeze the pesto to add the flavor of summer to winter dishes.

2 garlic cloves, halved
3 cups well-packed fresh basil leaves, stems removed and spun very dry
½ cup pine nuts
¾ teaspoon salt
¼ teaspoon freshly ground black pepper
½ to ⅔ cup extra virgin or regular olive oil
⅓ cup freshly grated Parmesan cheese

With the motor running, toss the garlic down the feed tube of a food processor to mince it. Add the basil, pine nuts, salt, and pepper; process until very finely chopped.

With the motor running, add oil in a thin stream until the mixture is thick but not runny. Stop the motor once or twice to scrape down the bottom and sides of the bowl with a rubber spatula.

Stir in the cheese. Transfer the pesto to a jar and pour a thin layer of oil on top to preserve the color. Cover and refrigerate until needed. The pesto will keep up to 7 days.

For longer storage, spray an ice-cube tray with nonstick cooking spray. Fill with pesto. When they are solidly frozen, transfer the pesto cubes to a plastic freezer bag or container.

Makes about 1 cup.

VARIATION

Parsley-Walnut Pesto

Follow the recipe for Basil Pesto, substituting fresh flat-leaf parsley for the basil and walnuts for the pine nuts. Omit the cheese.

To avoid a bitter taste, blanch the walnuts: Put them into a saucepan with water to cover. Bring to a boil, drain, and rinse. When the nuts are dry, toast them lightly in a small dry skillet.

Makes about 1 cup.

Cannellini Beans

Leftover cooked dried beans can be frozen and used in soups or casseroles.

    1 cup dried cannellini (white kidney beans), picked over and rinsed
    1 tablespoon olive oil
    1 large yellow onion, chopped
    1 garlic clove, chopped
    4 cups water
    ½ to ¾ teaspoon salt
    3 (2-inch) sprigs fresh rosemary or ¼ teaspoon dried
       Freshly ground black pepper

Soak the beans in 6 cups of water overnight in a cool place. The next day drain and rinse the beans. (If you forget to do this, there's a second option: Bring the beans to a boil, cook 2 minutes. Remove from the heat and let them stand 1 hour. Drain and rinse. Proceed as follows.)

Heat the oil in the same pot over medium heat and sauté the onion and garlic until they're sizzling and fragrant, 3 minutes. Add the beans and the 4 cups of water. Simmer the beans, with lid barely ajar, until they are tender, about 1 hour. Add the salt and rosemary and cook 5 minutes more. Add pepper to your taste.

Serve the beans with some of their cooking liquid or use them, drained, in recipes.

Makes about 4 cups.

VARIATIONS

Dried Beans, Simply Simmered

Many kinds of dried beans can be cooked by simmering on the rangetop. Follow the preceding recipe, omitting rosemary and varying the herbs as you wish. If desired, omit garlic. Cooking time depends on the kind of bean and its age: from 1 hour to 2 hours, more for chick-peas or soybeans. Taste is the best test.

Here are some seasoning combinations:

Pink beans: 1 tablespoon chopped fresh marjoram or 1 teaspoon dried

Pinto beans: 1 tablespoon chopped fresh cilantro or 1 teaspoon dried

Red kidney beans or *black-eyed peas:* 1 tablespoon chopped fresh summer savory or 1 teaspoon dried

Chick-peas: A few leaves of chopped fresh sage or 1 to 2 hot dried red peppers

Adzuki beans: 1 tablespoon minced fresh ginger sautéed with the onion

Black beans: 2 teaspoons chopped fresh thyme or ½ teaspoon dried, or thin slivers of orange peel

Roman beans or *soybeans:* Add 1 cup chopped tomatoes with the water; 1 tablespoon chopped fresh oregano or ½ teaspoon dried makes a complementary addition.

Zesty Fresh Tomato Salsa

Serve this salsa as an accompaniment to enliven a dish of beans, savory corn pancakes, or any plainly cooked meat or fish.

2 cups seeded, chopped fresh plum tomatoes
1 seeded, diced mild green chile
1 to 2 seeded, minced fresh jalapeño chiles (see Note, page 120)
½ cup diced red or Vidalia onion
1 garlic clove, pressed through a garlic press
¼ cup fresh lime juice or red wine vinegar
2 tablespoons canola oil
2 tablespoons minced fresh cilantro or flat-leaf parsley
½ teaspoon salt
¼ teaspoon freshly ground black pepper

Combine all ingredients, cover, and chill several hours or overnight to blend flavors. Stir two or three times while chilling.

Makes about 3 cups.

Vegetable Stock

This flavorful, all-purpose soup stock is perfect for vegetarian dishes.

 2 tablespoons olive oil
 3 large leeks (1 bunch), well-rinsed and chopped
 2 onions, chopped
 3 garlic cloves, finely chopped
 4 celery stalks with leaves, chopped
 2 large carrots, chopped
 1 green bell pepper, seeded and chopped
10 cups water
 1 teaspoon chopped fresh thyme
    Several sprigs of fresh parsley, chopped
½ teaspoon salt
⅛ to ¼ teaspoon pepper

Heat the oil in a large pot. Add the leeks, onions, garlic, celery, carrots, and bell pepper. "Sweat" the vegetables over very low heat until they are lightly colored (not browned), 15 to 20 minutes. Add the water, thyme, parsley, and salt. Simmer, with lid barely ajar, 1 hour. Stir in the pepper.

Strain before using, pressing on vegetables with the back of a spoon. Discard vegetables.

Makes about 8 cups.

NOTE
Stock can be frozen for longer storage; 8-ounce containers are a convenient size.

Mediterranean Vegetable Stock

Another savory soup stock for vegetarian dishes.

2 tablespoons olive oil
2 onions, chopped
½ cup chopped shallots
1 bunch scallions with tops, chopped
3 garlic cloves, finely chopped
4 celery stalks with leaves, chopped
2 large carrots, chopped
1 red bell pepper, seeded and chopped
8 cups water
1 (14- to 16-oz.) can chopped tomatoes with juice
1 tablespoon chopped fresh basil
1 teaspoon chopped fresh tarragon or marjoram
   Several sprigs of fresh parsley, chopped
½ teaspoon salt
⅛ to ¼ teaspoon pepper

Heat the oil in a large pot. Add the onions, shallots, scallions, garlic, celery, carrots, and bell pepper. "Sweat" the vegetables over very low heat until they are lightly colored (not browned), 15 to 20 minutes. Add the water, tomatoes, basil, tarragon, parsley, and salt. Simmer, with lid barely ajar, 1 hour. Stir in the pepper.

Strain before using, pressing on vegetables with the back of a spoon. Discard vegetables.

Makes about 8 cups.

NOTE

Stock can be frozen for longer storage; 8-ounce containers are a convenient size.

Chicken-Mushroom Stock

A flavorful soup stock with a bonus of immunity-enhancing shiitake mushrooms. This is not a discard-the-solids stock, but a thrifty way to have your stock and some lovely boiled chicken for salad, too.

- 1 ounce dried shiitake mushrooms
- 3 pounds split chicken quarters, with bones, skinned
- 1 tablespoon olive oil
- 2 large onions, chopped
- 2 celery stalks with leaves, chopped
- 1 teaspoon *each* chopped fresh thyme, rosemary, and tarragon or ½ teaspoon dried herbs
- 8 cups water
- Several sprigs of fresh parsley or cilantro, chopped
- ½ teaspoon salt
- 2 large carrots, scraped and each cut into 2 pieces
- ⅛ to ¼ teaspoon pepper or to taste

Soak the mushrooms in hot water about 30 minutes. Strain the liquid through a paper coffee filter and reserve it. Chop the mushrooms.

Rinse the chicken in salted cold water; rinse and drain.

Heat the oil in a large pot. Add the onions and celery, and "sweat" the vegetables over very low heat until lightly colored, 10 minutes. Add the thyme, rosemary, and tarragon and cook 1 minute. Remove the vegetables and set aside. Using the same pot, lightly brown the chicken pieces over medium-high heat.

Return the vegetables to the pot. Add the water, mushrooms, reserved soaking liquid, parsley, and salt and simmer the broth, covered, 40 minutes. Add the carrots and pepper; cook 10 to 15 minutes.

Reserve the chicken and carrots for another use. Extra chicken can be frozen, moistened with a little broth. Strain the remaining stock and discard the remaining cooked vegetables.

Makes 8 cups.

NOTE

Stock can be frozen for longer storage; 8-ounce containers are a convenient size.

Yogurt Cheese

Use all-natural yogurt without gelatin or other stabilizers, such as pectin or gums, or the yogurt will not drain and thicken. Check the ingredient list carefully.

2　cups nonfat plain yogurt

Fit a large fine-meshed strainer with a paper coffee filter. Spoon the yogurt into the filter. Cover with plastic wrap and allow the yogurt to drain overnight in the refrigerator.

The next day, remove the cheese from the strainer and refrigerate it in a glass container. Discard the liquid whey or use it for soup.

Makes 1 cup.

VARIATIONS

Herbed-Pepper Cheese

Mix 1 cup yogurt cheese with 1 teaspoon chopped fresh thyme, 1 teaspoon chopped fresh savory or tarragon, 1 teaspoon chopped fresh basil, and ¼ teaspoon Spicy Mixed Pepper (opposite). Cover and chill for several hours to blend flavors. Bring to room temperature before serving. Serve with crackers.

Garlic Cheese

Mix 1 cup yogurt cheese with 1 clove garlic, pressed through a garlic press, ¼ teaspoon freshly ground white pepper, ¼ teaspoon celery salt, and ¼ teaspoon dried dill weed. Cover and chill for several hours to blend flavors. Bring to room temperature before serving. Serve with cocktail rye bread.

Olive Spread

Mix 1 cup yogurt cheese with ⅓ cup finely chopped pitted ripe olives and ⅓ cup fincly chopped stuffed green olives. Cover and chill for several hours to blend flavors. Bring to room temperature before serving. Serve with thinly sliced French bread.

Pineapple-Date Cheese

Mix 1 cup yogurt cheese with ½ cup drained, canned crushed pineapple and ½ cup finely chopped dates. Cover and chill for several hours to blend flavors. Bring to room temperature before serving. Serve with Boston brown bread.

Savory Clam Spread

Mix 1 cup yogurt cheese with 1 (6½-oz.) can drained chopped clams, 2 teaspoons Worcestershire sauce, and about ½ teaspoon hot pepper sauce or to taste. Cover and chill for several hours to blend flavors. Bring to room temperature before serving. Serve with crackers.

Spicy Mixed Pepper

If you enjoy a touch of spiciness, use this pepper in place of regular ground black pepper.

- 1 tablespoon ground black pepper
- 2 teaspoons ground white pepper
- 1 teaspoon ground cayenne pepper

Combine all ingredients very gently (to avoid sneezing) and store in a shaker.
Makes 2 tablespoons.

Boiled Shrimp

I think it's best to remove the shrimp shells after cooking, for two reasons. First, the shell preserves the flavor of the tender flesh. Second, many people are allergic to handling raw shrimp (I'm one of them), but it's safe to do so after cooking. I suggest wearing rubber gloves when working with raw shrimp.

1¼ pounds shrimp in shells
   Several lemon slices
 ½ bay leaf
 1 teaspoon salt
 ½ teaspoon whole peppercorns

Rinse the shrimp well. Combine all the ingredients in a saucepan and add water to cover. Bring the shrimp to a boil and simmer over very low heat 2 minutes. Remove the pan from the heat and let the shrimp stand in the hot liquid 5 to 10 minutes, until they have all turned bright pink.

Drain the shrimp. When they're cool enough to handle, peel off the shells. Remove the black vein that runs just under the skin along the curved back of the shrimp: Insert the point of a paring knife at the top (neck) and pull off the thin strip of flesh that covers the black vein. Sometimes the strip will come off in one piece and the vein with it. If not, cut a shallow channel to remove the vein.

Makes about 1 pound after shelling.

Vinaigrette

The favorite salad dressing of the Mediterranean region, it has many possible variations. The basic dressing can be stored at room temperature unless fresh ingredients are added.

⅓ cup red wine vinegar
½ teaspoon salt
¼ teaspoon freshly ground black pepper
¼ teaspoon dried basil, crushed
¼ teaspoon dried oregano or marjoram, crushed
⅔ cup extra-virgin olive oil

In a pint jar, mix the vinegar, salt, pepper, and herbs. Add the oil and shake well. Always shake the dressing well before drizzling on the salad.
Makes 1 cup.

VARIATIONS

Optional additions include minced garlic or shallots, fresh chopped parsley or dill, cayenne pepper, or a pinch of sugar. Such additions should be made about 1 hour before serving, to blend flavors. Once fresh ingredients are included, the dressing should be refrigerated.

Possible substitutions: lemon juice for all or part of the vinegar, white wine vinegar for red, pure olive oil for extra-virgin, or canola oil for part of the olive oil.

Sour Milk for Baking

Sour milk can replace buttermilk in many recipes for baked goods but not in salad dressings. This is a great convenience when you're inspired to bake and don't happen to have buttermilk in the refrigerator. The term sour milk *does not mean "spoiled milk," however, but fresh milk "soured" as follows.*

1 cup whole or low-fat milk
1 tablespoon white vinegar

Stir the vinegar into the milk and let stand at room temperature 15 minutes. Stir once. If less sour milk is needed, figure on 1 teaspoon vinegar for every ⅓ cup milk.
   Makes 1 cup.

Cinnamon Sugar

Before baking, shake a little cinnamon sugar on muffins or cakes you don't plan to frost or on hot toast.

2 tablespoons sugar
1 tablespoon ground cinnamon

Blend the sugar and cinnamon well. Store the mixture in a shaker.
Makes 3 tablespoons.

VARIATION

Ginger Sugar

Follow the preceding recipe, substituting ground ginger for cinnamon. This makes a lovely sweetener for tea as well as a flavorsome sprinkle for toast.

Bibliography

A list of books that describe the role nutrition plays in good health and successful aging and that provide recent scientific information on the foods featured in this cookbook.

Anderson, Jean, M.S., and Barbara Deskins, Ph.D., R.D. *The Nutrition Bible.* New York: William Morrow and Company, Inc., 1995

Bourre, Jean-Marie, M.D., translated from the French by Charles Ramble. *Brainfood.* Boston: Little, Brown and Company, 1993

Carper, Jean. *The Food Pharmacy.* New York: Bantam, 1989

Carper, Jean. *Stop Aging Now!* New York: HarperCollins, 1995

Castleman, Michael. *The Healing Herbs.* Emmaus, Pa.: Rodale Press, 1991

DeAngelis, Lissa, and Molly Siple. *Recipes for Change.* New York: Dutton, 1996

Hendler, Sheldon Saul, M.D., Ph.D. *The Doctors' Vitamin and Mineral Encyclopedia.* New York: Simon & Schuster, 1991

Herbert, Victor, M.D., F.A.C.P., and Genell J. Shbak-Sharpe, M.S. *The Mount Sinai School of Medicine Complete Book of Nutrition.* New York: St. Martin's Press, 1990

Kirschmann, Gayla J. and John D. *Nutrition Almanac, Fourth Edition.* New York: McGraw-Hill, 1996

Margen, Sheldon, M.D. *The Wellness Encyclopedia of Food and Nutrition.* Berkeley, Calif.: Health Letter Associates, 1992 (distributed by Random House)

Pennington, Jean A. T. *Bowes & Church's Food Values of Portions Commonly Used, Sixteenth Edition.* Philadelphia:

J. B. Lippincott Company, 1994

Somer, Elizabeth, M.A., R.D. *Food & Mood.* New York: Henry Holt, 1995

U.S. Department of Agriculture. *Handbook of the Nutritional Value of Foods in Common Units.* New York: Dover Publications, Inc., 1986

Winter, Ruth, M.S. *A Consumer's Guide to Medicines in Foods.* New York: Crown Trade Paperbacks, 1995

Wurtman, Judith J., Ph.D., with Margaret Danbrot. *Managing Your Mind and Mood Through Food.* New York: Harper & Row, 1988

NEWSLETTERS

A list of the newsletters that translate current medical research into layman's terms and are excellent sources of up-to-the-minute information on the link between nutrition and optimum health in later years. Some are solely devoted to nutrition; others contain general health information as well.

Consumer Reports on Health, 101 Truman Avenue, Yonkers, NY 10703-1057

Harvard Health Letter, P.O. Box 380, Boston, MA 02117

Health News, Massachusetts Medical Society (publishers of *The New England Journal of Medicine*), 1440 Main Street, Waltham, MA 02154-1649

Health After 50, 550 North Broadway, Suite 1100, Johns Hopkins, Baltimore, MD 21205-2001

Lifetime Health Letter, The University of Texas-Houston Health Science Center, 7000 Fannin, DCT 1212, Houston, TX 77030

Nutrition Action Healthletter, Center for Science in the Public Interest, Suite 300, 1875 Connecticut Avenue N.W., Washington, DC 20009-5728

Tufts University Health & Nutrition Letter, 53 Park Place, New York, NY 10007

University of California at Berkeley Wellness Letter, Health Letter Associates, P.O. Box 412, Prince Street Station, New York, NY 10012-0007

Women's Health Watch, Harvard Medical School Health Publications Group, 164 Longwood Avenue, Boston, MA 02115

Metric Conversion Charts

COMPARISON TO METRIC MEASURE

When you know	Symbol	Multiply by	To find	Symbol
teaspoons	tsp.	5.0	milliliters	ml
tablespoons	tbsp.	15.0	milliliters	ml
fluid ounces	fl. oz.	30.0	milliliters	ml
cups	c	0.24	liters	l
pints	pt.	0.47	liters	l
quarts	qt.	0.95	liters	l
ounces	oz.	28.0	grams	g
pounds	lb.	0.45	kilograms	kg
Fahrenheit	F	$^5/_9$(after subtracting 32)	Celsius	C

FAHRENHEIT TO CELSIUS

F	C
200–205	95
220–225	105
245–250	120
275	135
300–305	150
325–330	165
345–350	175
370–375	190
400–405	205
425–430	220
445–450	230
470–475	245
500	260

LIQUID MEASURE TO MILLILITERS

¼	teaspoon	=	1.25	milliliters
½	teaspoon	=	2.5	milliliters
¾	teaspoon	=	3.75	milliliters
1	teaspoon	=	5.0	milliliters
1¼	teaspoons	=	6.25	milliliters
1½	teaspoons	=	7.5	milliliters
1¾	teaspoons	=	8.75	milliliters
2	teaspoons	=	10.0	milliliters
1	tablespoon	=	15.0	milliliters
2	tablespoons	=	30.0	milliliters

LIQUID MEASURE TO LITERS

¼	cup	=	0.06	liters
½	cup	=	0.12	liters
¾	cup	=	0.18	liters
1	cup	=	0.24	liters
1¼	cups	=	0.3	liters
1½	cups	=	0.36	liters
2	cups	=	0.48	liters
2½	cups	=	0.6	liters
3	cups	=	0.72	liters
3½	cups	=	0.84	liters
4	cups	=	0.96	liters
4½	cups	=	1.08	liters
5	cups	=	1.2	liters
5½	cups	=	1.32	liters

Index